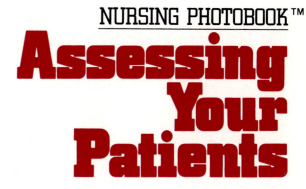

NURSING PHOTOBOOK™

Assessing Your Patients

NURSING82 BOOKS
INTERMED COMMUNICATIONS, INC.
SPRINGHOUSE, PENNSYLVANIA

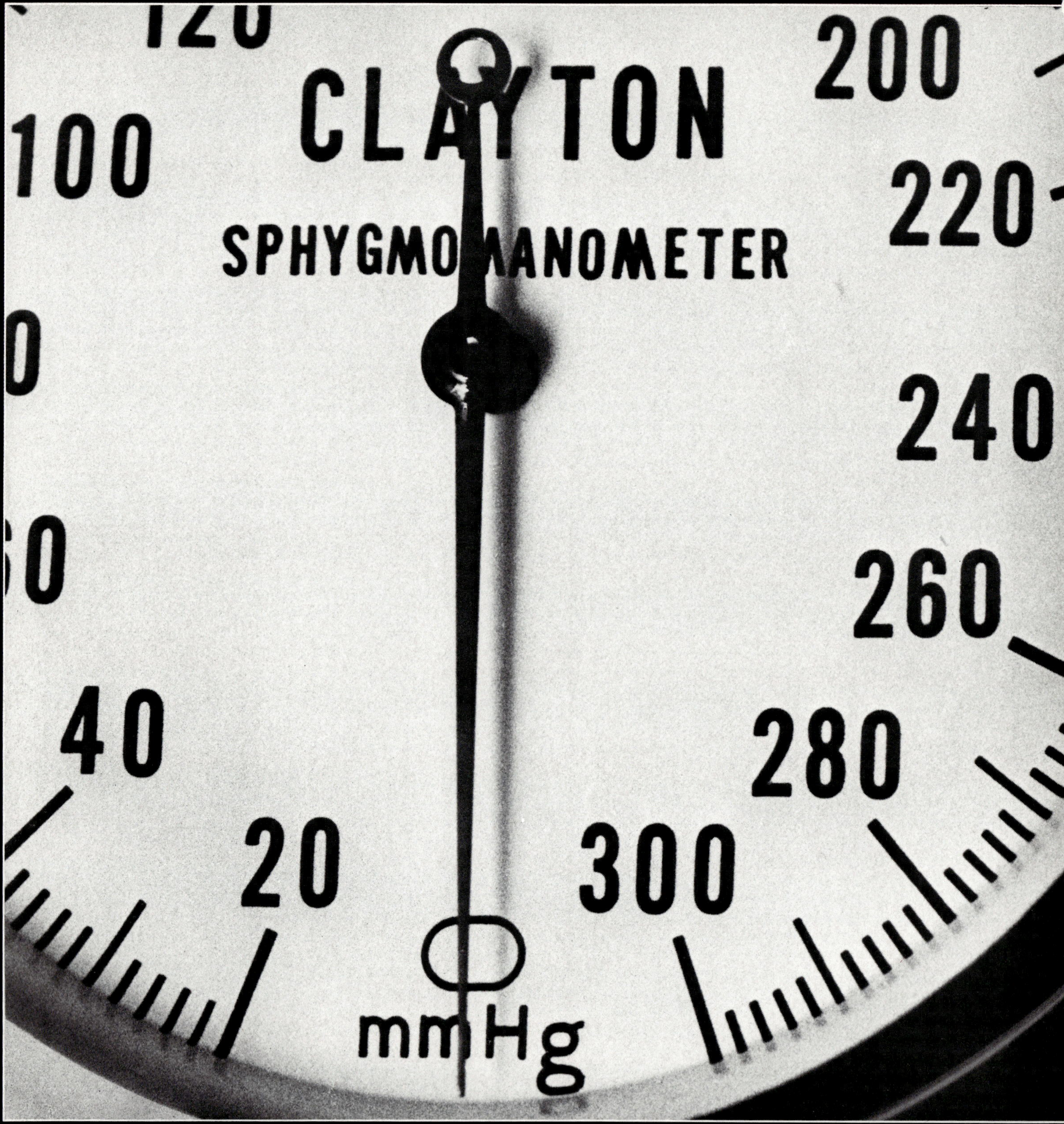
CLAYTON
SPHYGMOMANOMETER
mmHg
20
40
100
120
200
220
240
260
280
300

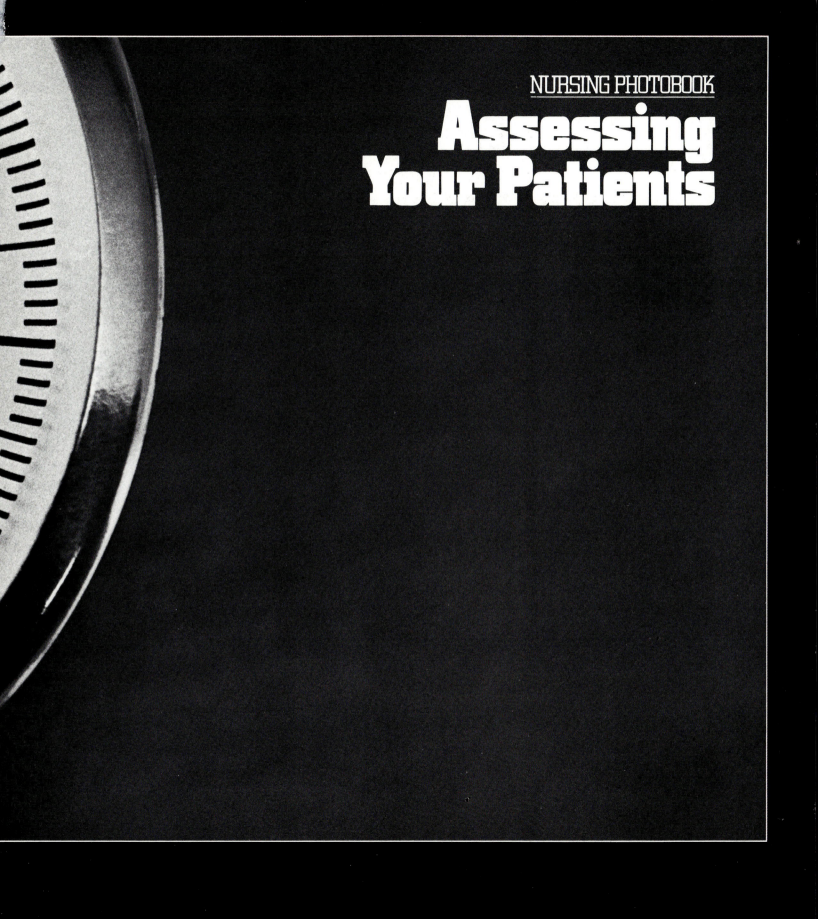

Assessing Your Patients

NURSING82 BOOKS

NURSING PHOTOBOOK™ SERIES
Providing Respiratory Care
Managing I.V. Therapy
Dealing with Emergencies
Giving Medications
Assessing Your Patients
Using Monitors
Providing Early Mobility
Giving Cardiac Care
Performing GI Procedures
Implementing Urologic Procedures
Controlling Infection
Ensuring Intensive Care
Coping with Neurologic Disorders
Caring for Surgical Patients
Working with Orthopedic Patients
Nursing Pediatric Patients
Helping Geriatric Patients
Attending Ob/Gyn Patients
Aiding Ambulatory Patients
Carrying Out Special Procedures

NURSING SKILLBOOK® SERIES
Reading EKGs Correctly
Dealing with Death and Dying
Managing Diabetics Properly
Assessing Vital Functions Accurately
Helping Cancer Patients Effectively
Giving Cardiovascular Drugs Safely
Giving Emergency Care Competently
Monitoring Fluid and Electrolytes Precisely
Documenting Patient Care Responsibly
Combatting Cardiovascular Diseases Skillfully
Coping with Neurologic Problems Proficiently
Using Crisis Intervention Wisely
Nursing Critically Ill Patients Confidently

NURSE'S REFERENCE LIBRARY™
Diseases
Diagnostics
Drugs
Assessment

Nursing82 **DRUG HANDBOOK™**

PROFESSIONAL GUIDE TO DRUGS™
PROFESSIONAL GUIDE TO DISEASES™

NURSING PHOTOBOOK™ SERIES
PUBLISHER
Eugene W. Jackson

EDITORIAL DIRECTOR
Jean Robinson

CLINICAL DIRECTOR
Barbara McVan, RN

ART DIRECTOR
Lisa A. Gilde

Intermed Communications
Book Division
DIRECTOR
Timothy B. King

DIRECTOR, RESEARCH
Elizabeth O'Brien

DIRECTOR, PRODUCTION AND PURCHASING
Bacil Guiley

Staff for this volume
BOOK EDITOR
Patricia Reilly Urosevich

CLINICAL EDITOR
Mary Horstman Obenrader, RN

ASSOCIATE EDITOR
Jean Patterson

PHOTOGRAPHER
Paul A. Cohen

ASSOCIATE DESIGNERS
Linda Jovinelly Franklin
Carol Stickles

CLINICAL EDITORIAL ASSOCIATE
Mary Gyetvan, RN, BSEd

EDITORIAL/GRAPHIC COORDINATOR
Doreen K. Stowers

COPY EDITOR
Barbara Hodgson

EDITORIAL STAFF ASSISTANT
Evelyn M. James

ASSISTANT PHOTOGRAPHER
Thomas Staudenmayer

DARKROOM ASSISTANTS
James M. Davidson
Gary Donnelly

ART PRODUCTION MANAGER
Wilbur D. Davidson

ARTISTS
Lorraine Carbo
Darcy Feralio
Diane Fox
Robert Perry
Sandra Simms
Louise Stamper

RESEARCHER
Vonda Heller

TYPOGRAPHY MANAGER
David C. Kosten

TYPOGRAPHY ASSISTANTS
Ethel Halle
Diane Paluba

PRODUCTION MANAGER
Robert L. Dean, Jr.

ASSISTANT PRODUCTION MANAGER
Deborah C. Meiris

PRODUCTION ASSISTANT
M. Eileen Hunsicker

ILLUSTRATORS
Dimitrios N. Bastas
Jack Crane
Jean Gardner
Tom Herbert
Robert Jackson
Cynthia Mason
John R. Murphy
Bud Yingling

SERIES GRAPHIC DESIGNER
John C. Isely

COVER PHOTO
Seymour Mednick

Clinical consultants
for this volume
Catherine L. Gilliss, RN, BSN, MSN, ANP
Assistant Professor
School of Nursing, University of Portland
Portland, Oregon

Joyce K. Shoemaker, RN, BSN, MSN
Vice Chairman, Nursing Department
College of Allied Health Professions
Temple University
Philadelphia, Pennsylvania

Copyright © 1982, 1980 by Intermed
Communications, Inc.,
1111 Bethlehem Pike, Springhouse, Pa. 19477
All rights reserved. Reproduction in
whole or part by any means
whatsoever without written permission
of the publisher is prohibited by law.
Printed in the United States of America.
041082

Library of Congress Cataloging in Publication Data

Main entry under title:

Assessing your patients.

(Nursing80 Photobook)
Bibliography: p.
Includes index.
1. Physical diagnosis—Atlases. 2. Nursing—Atlases.
3. Medical history taking.
[DNLM: 1. Diagnosis—Nursing texts. 2. Nursing process.
WY100 A846]
RT48.A86   616.07'54'023613   80-36819
ISBN 0-916730-24-7

Contents

Contributors

At the time of original publication, these contributors held the following positions.

Julie F. Boyle earned her BSN degree at Georgetown University, Washington, D.C. She is assistant head nurse of the spinal cord injury (SCI) unit and coordinator of the SCI and GU departments at James A. Haley VA Medical Center, Tampa, Fla.

Catherine L. Gilliss, one of the advisers on this book, is an assistant professor at the University of Portland (Ore.) School of Nursing. She has a BSN degree from Duke University in Durham, N.C., and an MSN degree from The Catholic University of America, Washington, D.C. She earned ANP (Adult Nurse Practitioner) certification from the University of Rochester, in New York. Ms. Gilliss is a doctoral candidate at the University of California School of Nursing in San Francisco.

Maryann Hall, 1st Lieutenant, U.S. Air Force Nursing Corps, is a staff nurse at Wilford Hall Medical Center, Lackland Air Force Base, San Antonio, Tex. A graduate of Philadelphia (Pa.) General Hospital, she also attended Temple University, Philadelphia, and San Antonio (Tex.) College. The manuscript submitted by Lieutenant Hall reflects her private views and should not be considered as an official view of the U.S. Air Force or Department of Defense.

Jane Irvin-Pethick, a graduate of Wagner College School of Nursing, Staten Island, N.Y., earned an MSN degree and CNM (Certified Nurse Midwife) certification at the University of Utah College of Nursing in Salt Lake City. Ms. Irvin-Pethick is nursing supervisor at Montgomery Hospital, Norristown, Pa.

Karen Lieberman is a graduate of Montgomery College School of Nursing, Takoma Park, Md. She is head nurse of the coronary care unit at Metropolitan Hospital, Philadelphia, Pa.

Rosemary Noone McCormick holds a BSN degree from Wilkes College, Wilkes Barre, Pa. She also completed a nurse internship program at Massachusetts General Hospital in Boston. Ms. McCormick is a psychiatric charge nurse at Kirksville (Mo.) Osteopathic Hospital.

Charlotte L. Noesgaard is a nursing faculty member at Vanier College, Montreal, Quebec, Canada. A graduate of Royal Alexandra School of Nursing, Edmonton, Alberta, she earned a BN degree at McGill University, Montreal.

Joyce K. Shoemaker, also an adviser on this book, earned BSN and MSN degrees at the University of Pennsylvania, Philadelphia. She is a doctoral candidate at Columbia University Teachers College in New York City. Ms. Shoemaker is vice chairman of the department of nursing at Temple University College of Allied Health Professions in Philadelphia.

Cheryl A. Walker is an instructor at the University of Colorado School of Medicine, department of medicine, division of internal medicine, department of family practice. A graduate of the University of Florida in Gainesville, she earned an MN degree at the University of Washington in Seattle, and CNP (Certified Nurse Practitioner) certification from Emory University, Atlanta, Ga. Ms. Walker belongs to the American Nurses' Association, and the Council of Primary Care Nurse Practitioners.

Introduction

If you think patient assessment isn't a critical part of the nursing process, think again. Whether you work in a hospital, a public health center, a clinic, or a doctor's office, the nursing decisions and judgments you make will be based on your initial and ongoing assessments.

How do you ensure accurate and effective patient assessment? Understanding the basics isn't enough. You'll need to perfect the skills of interviewing, observing, and inspecting. You'll want to know exactly what to look for and how to evaluate your findings.

We at NURSING BOOKS are aware of your responsibilities and want to help. That's why we've put together this PHOTOBOOK—to *show* you how to assess a patient properly. Examine it carefully. Let the clearly written text, photographs, and illustrations guide you through a complete head-to-toe assessment.

What are some of the features that make this PHOTOBOOK so valuable? For starters, it offers practical advice from working nurses, who know the special techniques you must master to do a proper assessment. As an example, do you know how to grade a heart murmur correctly? This PHOTOBOOK will show you. It'll also show you how to perform an Allen's test, how to percuss and palpate your patient's sinuses, and how to test and evaluate cranial nerve function.

Everything else you need to know about patient assessment is included too; for example, illustrated charts showing you how to identify and evaluate common abnormalities, full-color illustrations to help you locate anatomical landmarks, and lists of sample questions to ask your patient about his body systems.

Patient assessment. What better way to perfect your skills in this area than to study this PHOTOBOOK. Our clinical staff, editors, advisers, and contributors have checked and rechecked the information included to make certain it's accurate and up to date. Use this PHOTOBOOK as a tool. You'll benefit, and so will your patients.

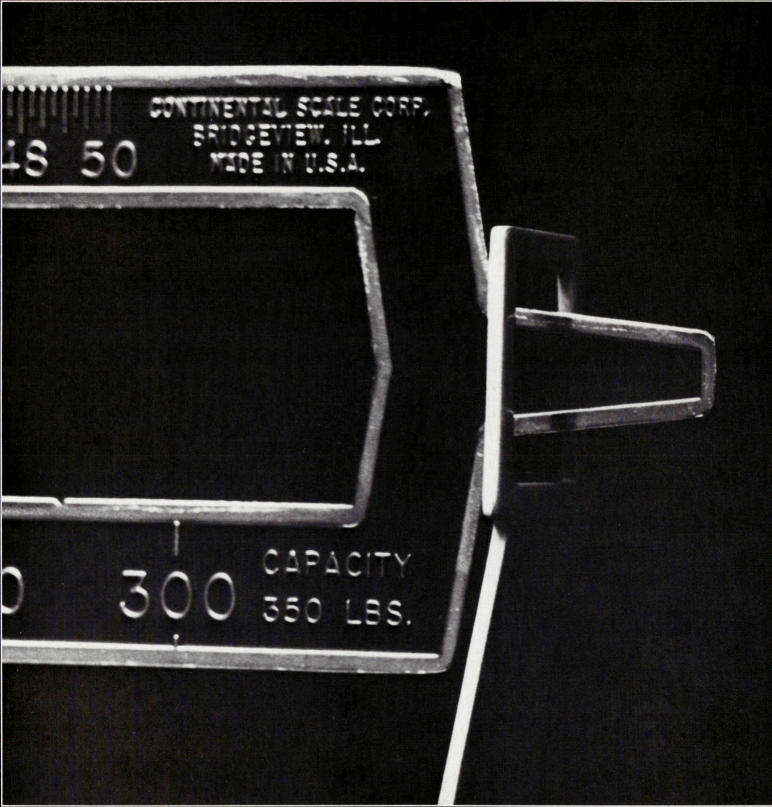

Viewing Your Whole Patient

Interview

Preliminary examination

Interview

No doubt you're aware how important it is to perform a good patient assessment. As you know, you'll collect data for your patient's assessment by using your skills of interviewing, inspection, and observation.

But do you know how to interview your patient effectively? Do you know how to prepare the environment so the interview will proceed smoothly? Suppose your patient speaks another language, is unconscious or forgetful. Suppose he's uncooperative and won't answer your questions.

How does assessment fit into the nursing process? Do you know what a nursing diagnosis is?

Learning how to understand and cope with these problems is your responsibility. We can help you meet that responsibility with the information on the following pages.

Assessment; The foundation of the nursing process

How does patient assessment fit into the nursing process? To know the correct answer, you must first understand what the nursing process is: a systematic method of problem-solving through continuous patient assessment. Before you can provide quality care for your patients, you must first be able to identify and solve their problems. Your initial assessment lays the foundation for problem-solving, as you can see in this chart of the nursing process.

Step 1. Recognize problems
Observe and document your patient's problems and needs. This step forms the foundation of the nursing process. The information you collect by properly interviewing and examining your patient gives you a data base on which to build his care plan.

Step 2. Define
Clearly identify—or define—your patient's problems and needs. By defining the problems you've discovered in your initial assessment, you'll be better able to plan his care.
Remember, defining a patient's problem is *not* the same as defining its *cause*, which, of course, is the doctor's responsibility. You simply list the patient's problems and needs as you know they exist. When you do, include his personal needs—for example, financial and emotional—as well as his physical ones.

Step 3. Plan
Devise possible solutions to the problems and needs you've defined in your patient assessment. Doing so will help you plan, write, direct, implement, and evaluate an individualized patient care plan. A well-written care plan eases communication between shifts and assures your patient continuity of care.

Step 4. Implement
Put your solutions to work. In this step of the nursing process, you're implementing the specific instructions outlined in your patient's care plan. You'll also be documenting what you've done, as well as assessing your patient's progress (or lack of it).

Step 5. Evaluate
Finally, evaluate how effective your solutions have been in solving your patient's problems. To do this, check his care plan against his progress notes. Were the instructions carried out? Were they effective? If not, you'll need to reassess your patient's problems, come up with other solutions, and revise his care plan to include them.
Quality patient care is what you accomplish by using the nursing process to assess and reassess your patient's problems, needs, and progress.

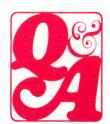

Your nursing diagnosis: What is it?

Have you ever asked yourself this question? What's the difference between a nursing diagnosis and a medical diagnosis?

Well, here's the answer. As you interview, observe, and inspect your patient, you're collecting data that focuses on his problems and needs as *you* know they exist. You're also attempting to discover how he perceives these problems and needs. Putting this information together allows you to identify his problems, which, as you know, is the same as making a nursing diagnosis.

How does this differ from a medical diagnosis? When you make a nursing diagnosis, you'll simply *identify the patient's problems*. The doctor's medical diagnosis attempts to *identify the cause* of the patient's problems. The data the doctor collects will aid in treating your patient's symptoms.

Interview

Six rules for effective interviewing

As you know, doing a complete and thorough initial assessment of your patient can help you cope with his problems and needs. But learning how to interview effectively requires skill and practice. Perfect your technique by following these six rules carefully.

1
Create a pleasant interviewing atmosphere.

First, evaluate the lighting. Is it adequate? Too much or too little light will cause eye strain and fatigue for you and your patient.

Will noise prevent you or your patient from concentrating on the questions? If you can't eliminate it, consider moving to a quieter place or rescheduling the interview.

Is the interviewing area private? Your patient may not express himself freely if he feels he's being overheard. If possible, try to schedule the interview when his roommate isn't present. Ask visitors to step out in the hall temporarily. But allow your patient to have a friend or family member present, if he requests it.

Is your patient ready to be interviewed? If he's tired, apprehensive, or in pain, he'll be too upset to provide you with information. Reschedule the interview. If your patient's in pain, try to obtain a doctor's order for pain medication.

Allow 15 minutes or more for the interview. Don't rush; an effective interview may take as long as an hour. Suppose you don't have that much time to spend uninterrupted. Schedule several short interviews, and explain to your patient why you're doing so.

2
Gather all available information about your patient before you interview him.

Get as much information as possible from admission forms and previous hospital records (if any). Doing so will save you time and will avoid annoying and tiring your patient. However, always quickly review admission information with your patient during the interview. He may have been so confused and upset on admission that he gave incorrect or incomplete information.

Make sure you have your patient's correct address, age, occupation, and other vital statistics. These facts can relate directly to your patient's condition. For example, if your patient works in a chemical factory, he may have health problems related to chemical exposure. Or if your patient has inadequate housing, some of his problems may result from a poor heating system or unsanitary living conditions.

3
Try to develop a good rapport with your patient.

Before you begin the interview, sit at eye level and talk to your patient for a few minutes. If you stand, he may feel rushed and may cut his answers short or omit important information.

Show a genuine interest in what your patient is telling you. Maintaining eye contact and occasionally repeating what he's told you can help you do this. However, if you seem abrupt, preoccupied, or disinterested, he probably won't confide in you.

Explain the purpose of the interview to your patient, so he understands how he benefits from it. Stress the need for his cooperation and honesty. Give him examples of how the information he gives you can help you plan his care.

4
Set the tone for the interview.

Begin your interview by asking, "How do you feel?" or, "What's been troubling you the most?" Allowing your patient to talk about his chief complaint can alert you to specific signs and symptoms you should investigate. It can also help you assess your patient's emotional state and level of understanding.

Keep the interview informal yet professional. Let your patient answer your questions leisurely, but if he gets too far off the track, lead him back to the subject. To do this tactfully, ask him a question that reminds him of his chief complaint, such as, "Can you tell me more about the pain in your legs?"

During the interview, be sure to speak clearly and simply. Avoid using medical terminology. Your patient may be reluctant to admit he doesn't understand the terms.

Not sure your patient comprehends your questions? Ask him to repeat, in his own words, what you've said.

Pay close attention to what your patient says. Does he understand what's wrong with him? Does he seem frightened or apprehensive? Getting in touch with your patient's feelings in this way will help you reach him.

5
Form effective questions.

Try to ask questions that require more than a yes or no answer. You'll find examples of open-ended questions in each section of this PHOTOBOOK. Open-ended questioning keeps the interview focused on your patient's concerns and encourages him to give more complete answers.

When your patient alerts you to one of his problems by describing signs and symptoms, ask him to elaborate. Detailed descriptions are particularly important when your patient uses terminology you're unfamiliar with.

Listen closely to your patient's answers. They may suggest other questions to ask. For example, suppose you ask, "How is your sight?" If your patient replies, "My vision is sometimes blurry," continue this line of questioning. Ask: "How often does the blurring occur? How long have you had it?"

Dealing with interviewing problems

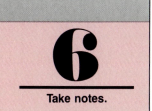

6

Take notes.

Don't try to document all the information you gather as you interview your patient. Instead, jot down dates, times, key words or phrases, and use them later to complete a patient history form for your patient's records. You'll find a sample of a properly completed form at the back of this book. Study it.

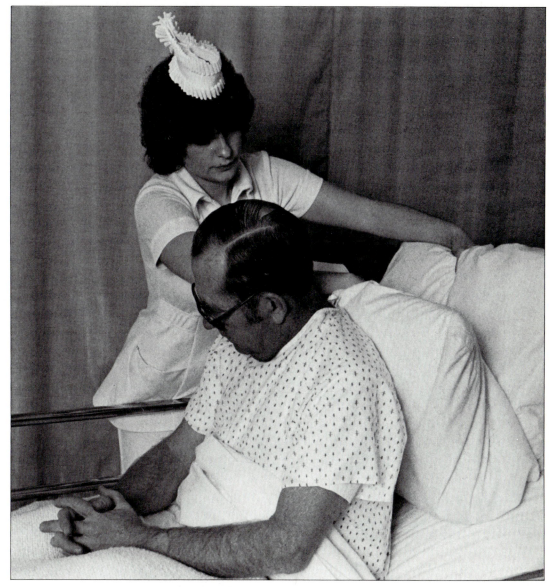

No matter how skilled you are at interviewing, you will occasionally face problems. Do you know how to cope with special challenges? Study the following case histories carefully for practical help.

Case 1: The uncooperative patient

Suppose you're interviewing Clarence Hawkins, a 54-year-old security guard. Mr. Hawkins answers your first few questions abruptly, then turns his head away and refuses to speak to you. What do you do?

First, find out why Mr. Hawkins isn't cooperating. Is he in pain or uncomfortable? If so, consult a doctor about pain medication for him. Try to make him more comfortable with an extra blanket or pillow. Give him a backrub or offer him something to drink. Do whatever you can to make him more at ease

Is he upset about his illness or personal problems? Empathize and encourage him to express himself. Once you know what's bothering him, you may be able to do something about it.

Make sure Mr. Hawkins knows why you need to interview him and how he'll benefit. He may be uncooperative because he thinks you're prying.

No matter what you do, Mr. Hawkins may not want to cooperate with you. Reschedule the interview, if you think he'll act differently later. But don't get discouraged. As you know, many people are reluctant to confide personal information to strangers. Be understanding. As you develop a rapport with Mr. Hawkins, he may become more friendly.

Note: If you continue to have problems, ask a coworker to try interviewing Mr. Hawkins for you. He or she may have more success.

Interview

Dealing with interviewing problems continued

Case 2: The forgetful patient

Imagine you're interviewing 74-year-old Eppie Weaver. Her admission form tells you that she's a retired registered nurse who's currently living in a nursing home. But Mrs. Weaver has trouble recalling such information and becomes increasingly agitated by further questions. How should you react?

Try to be calm and reassuring. If you become annoyed or impatient, you may make the situation worse, especially if your patient is sensitive about her poor memory. *Nursing tip:* You may be able to help Mrs. Weaver remember important facts by giving her a frame of reference. Help her relate the information you want to some important event in her life. For example, ask her questions like, "Was it before you were married? While your husband was in the armed forces? Did it happen before you had your first child?"

No matter how hard she tries, Mrs. Weaver may not recall certain facts. You may not have time to wait for her memory to improve. In such a case, ask Mrs. Weaver's permission to contact a family member or a friend to provide the information.

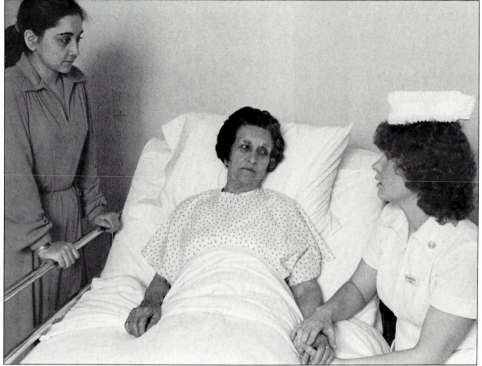

Case 3: The patient who speaks a foreign language

Katsuhiro Itoh has been admitted to your care with second-degree burns on his hands. Although he's no longer in pain, he seems withdrawn and frightened. When you approach him for a patient interview, you realize he speaks almost no English. How can you communicate with him?

Perhaps Katsuhiro has a friend or family member who is bilingual. Or maybe one of your coworkers can act as an interpreter. If you work in a hospital, call the social service director. She may have a list of coworkers who can help.

Keep foreign language phrase books at the nurses' desk so you can quickly translate common words and phrases. In a pinch, try sign language and pictures.

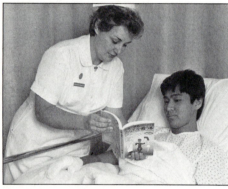

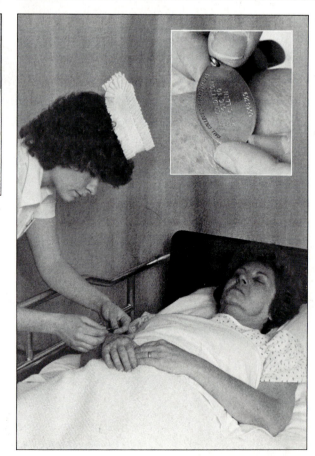

Case 4: The unconscious patient

Consider this situation. Violet Moretti is a 50-year-old housewife who's recently been admitted for a cerebrovascular accident (CVA). Although Mrs. Moretti is already receiving treatment in your unit, she's still unconscious. Even when she regains consciousness, she'll probably be too ill to answer your questions. How can you get the information you need to effectively plan nursing care?

If Mrs. Moretti arrived at the hospital in an ambulance, ask the attendant for information. Also, look for Medic Alert™ jewelry (see inset) or an Identa-Drug Wallet™. Consult Mrs. Moretti's family and friends. They can inform you about her medical history, family doctor, personality, likes, and dislikes.

Preliminary examination

You've interviewed your patient. Now, begin the thorough examination that's necessary to collect the data for your initial assessment. To examine your patient, you must carefully observe and inspect her. This process, of course, is an *ongoing* one that begins at your patient's admission and ends at her discharge.

On the next few pages, we'll show you how to perform a preliminary examination of your patient that'll help you spot possible problem areas to investigate more thoroughly later. We'll also show you how to palpate, percuss, and auscultate your patient correctly.

Make sure you understand the skills involved in this section before you read the rest of this book.

Performing a preliminary examination

1 *To set assessment priorities, get an overview of your patient's condition before you do a complete head-to-toe examination. Here's how:*

First, explain to your patient that you'll be doing a physical exam. Then, ask her to stand up, so you can observe her stature. If possible, measure her height, as the nurse is doing here. Check her posture. Does she stand erect, or is she slumped over? Is her spine straight, or does it have an unusual curve? How old does she look? Does she seem older or younger than the age recorded on her admission form?

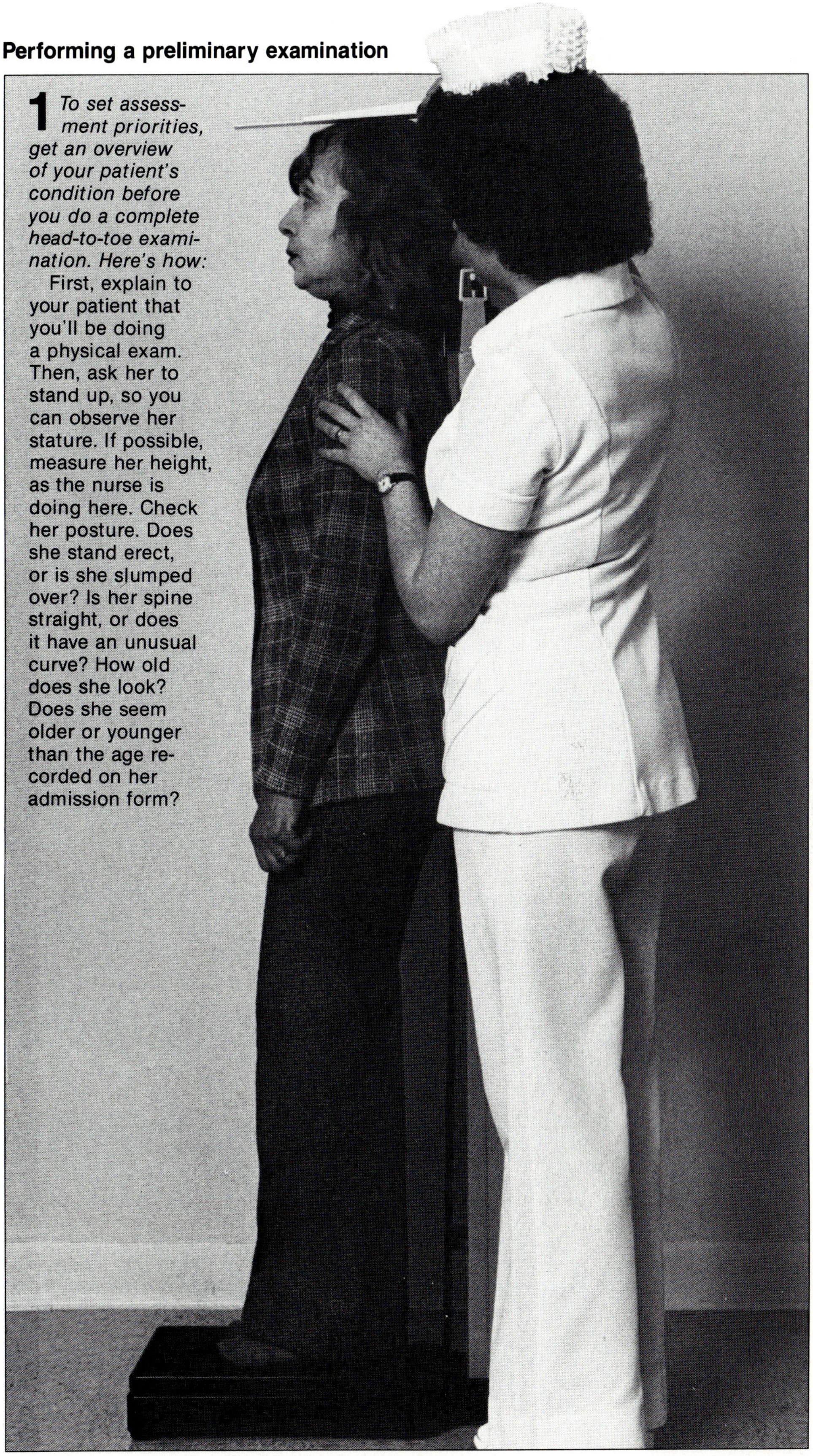

Preliminary examination

Performing a preliminary examination continued

2 Next, weigh your patient and assess her body size. Compare her height and weight to the averages on a chart.

Are her body proportions normal? Note the size of her trunk, arms, and legs. As you can see in this photo, the distance from the top of her head to her pubic symphysis should approximately equal the distance from her pubic symphysis to the bottom of her feet.

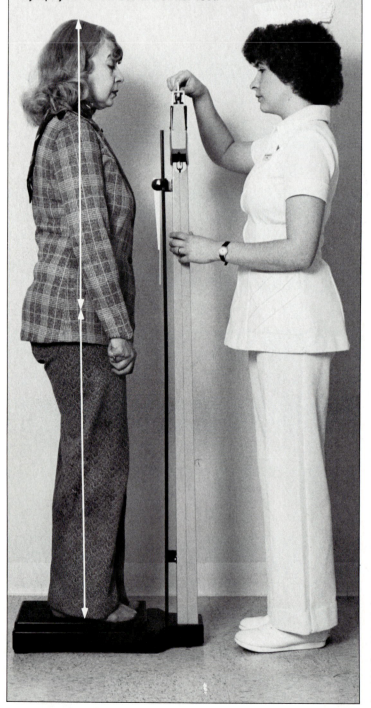

3 Now, ask your patient to walk across the room. Does she have a brisk gait? Does one foot drag? Check for any signs of unusual rapidity, slowness, uncoordination, paralysis, or spasticity.

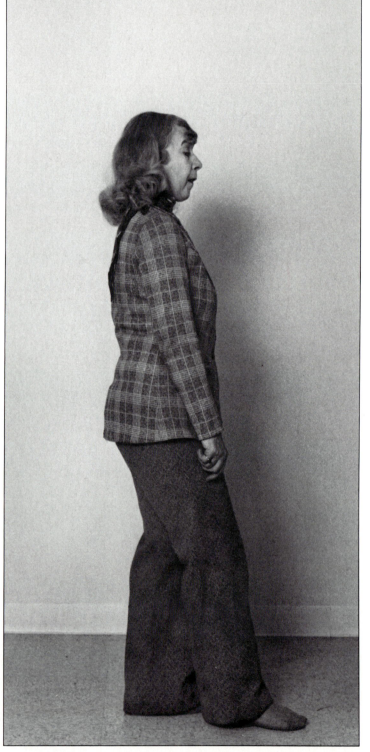

4 What about your patient's facial expression. Is it fixed? Or does it change in ways appropriate to the circumstances? Is she uncooperative, resentful, friendly, depressed, or angry? Is she unusually talkative or taciturn?

Note the pitch, pace, and clarity of her speech. Pay particular attention to her vocabulary and sentence structure. Does she speak coherently? Note any inability to form meaningful sentences, even though it may only reflect her socioeconomic state. Next, observe her general state of awareness. Does she have a short attention span? Is she alert? Or does she seem confused or preoccupied?

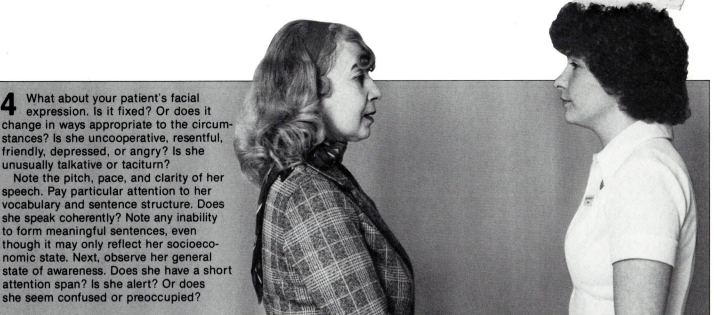

5 Now, get an impression of your patient's personal hygiene and grooming habits. Do her clothes fit properly? Are her nails clean? Can you detect any unusual odors; for example, alcohol, acetone, or urine?

Remember, environmental and cultural influences always have some effect on your patient's personal hygiene and grooming habits. But poor hygiene and personal neglect may also be caused by physical and mental disorders that need medical attention. They may even indicate abuse.

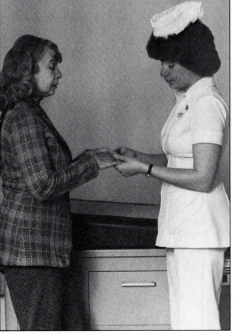

6 Prepare your patient for the complete head-to-toe examination you'll be doing later by instructing her to put on a gown. As you help her, observe any scars, cuts, bruises, or unusual skin colorations she may have.

Also, note how hair is distributed on your patient's body. Does it seem excessive, particularly in a woman or child?

Feel your patient's skin. Is it hot, dry, cool, or moist? You'll find details on how to document unusual skin conditions on page 21.

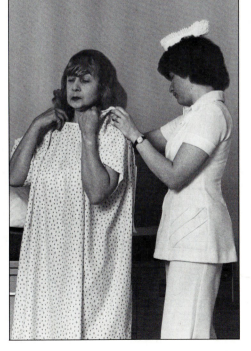

7 Now, ask your patient to sit on the exam table. Then, examine her arms. Does she have good movement in her shoulder and elbow joints? Are the bones straight? Does she have good muscle tone? Or do her muscles look atrophied?

[Inset] Ask your patient to grasp your hands and squeeze them. As she does, check her hands and wrists for coordination, muscle tone, strength, and appearance. Do they look swollen or seem stiff?

Are any fingers missing? Does she have good movement in her fingers and wrists?

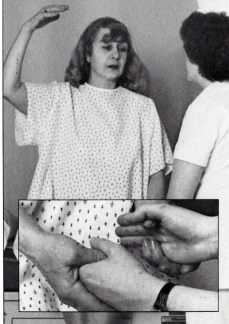

Preliminary examination

Performing a preliminary examination continued

8 Examine your patient's legs. Are they properly aligned? Or are the bones curved inward? Look for tissue and joint swelling (particularly in her ankles and knees), unusual skin rashes, cuts, distended or bluish veins.

Are both legs equal in length? Check the color and temperature of her feet. Are any toes missing? Look for tremors, ulcers, calluses, or scales.

[Inset] Finally, check your patient's legs, hips, and ankles for range of motion.

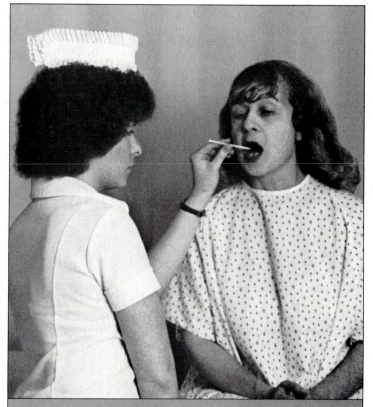

9 Next, take your patient's temperature. Use the oral method, if possible. If your patient is very young or can't hold a thermometer in her mouth, use the axillary or rectal methods.

Important: Before you take your patient's oral temperature, ask her if she's smoked or had anything to drink within the past 20 minutes. If she has, wait 15 minutes before taking her temperature.

To get an accurate oral reading, leave the thermometer in your patient's mouth for 8 to 9 minutes. To get an accurate rectal reading, leave the thermometer in your patient's rectum for at least 2½ minutes. Remember: If you use an electronic thermometer, leave the electronic probe in place until signaled by the machine. (You should see a light or hear a tone in approximately 30 seconds.)

The normal range for an oral temperature is 97.7° to 99.5° F. (36.5° to 37.5° C.). The normal range for a rectal temperature is 98.8° to 100.5° F. (37.1° to 38° C.). Normally, axillary temperature readings are from 96.7° to 98.5° F. (36° to 37° C.).

All temperature readings register 1° to 2° F. (.6° to 1.2° C.) lower in early morning than in late afternoon. A high reading may indicate infection, excitement, or exposure to an extremely hot environment. A subnormal temperature may be an indication of early shock.

Now, you're ready to begin a more detailed patient examination. Ensure accuracy by inspecting body parts in a systematic fashion: for example, from the patient's right side to the patient's left side, as shown in this PHOTOBOOK. Then, don't vary this method throughout the inspection.

How to palpate, percuss, and auscultate

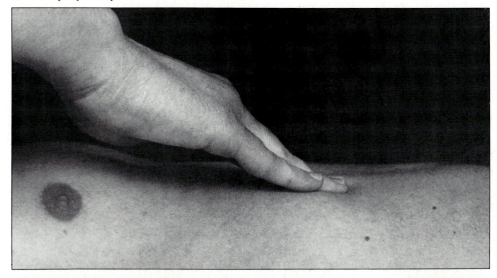

1 *Throughout this PHOTOBOOK, you'll be learning how to do a complete head-to-toe examination of your patient. Do you have the necessary skills to examine your patient properly? For example, do you know how to palpate, percuss, and auscultate? If not, read this photostory.*

In this photo, you see how to palpate correctly. Palpation will help you confirm data that you gather from observation.

Use light palpation (indenting your patient's skin about ½" [1.3 cm]) to check the temperature and moistness of the skin and to detect large tumors and tender or painful areas.

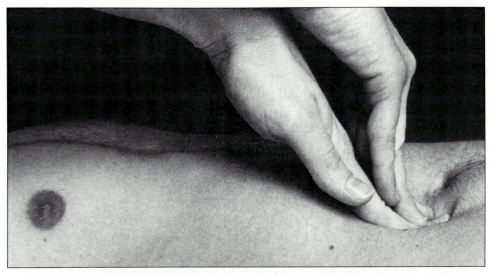

2 You'll use deep palpation (indenting your patient's skin *more* than ½" [1.3 cm]) to locate organs and determine their size, to check for spasticity or rigidity, to feel pulsations, to detect crepitus and tumors.

🖒 *Nursing tip:* To increase your fingertip pressure, place one hand on top of the other to palpate.

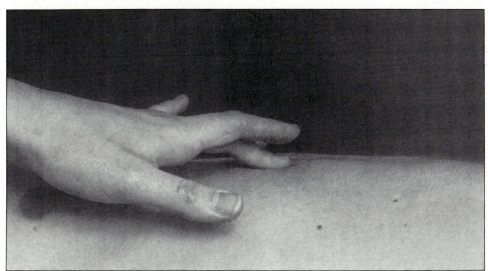

3 When you percuss your patient—and evaluate the sounds produced—you can determine the density, size, and location of underlying organs and structures. To percuss correctly, place the first joint of your left middle finger on your patient, as shown here. Keep the rest of your hand poised above the skin.

Preliminary examination

How to palpate, percuss, and auscultate continued

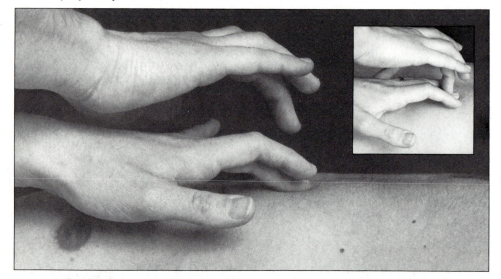

4 Make sure the fingers on your right hand are flexed and your wrist action is loose.

[Inset] Now, use your right middle finger to tap the left finger *exactly* as shown here. As soon as you've done this, withdraw your right finger, so you don't damp the vibration.

Tap several times, listening carefully. Then, move your hands slightly, and repeat the procedure at other points. Compare the difference in sounds (if any).

Important: Are you left-handed? Put your right middle finger on the patient, and tap with your left middle finger.

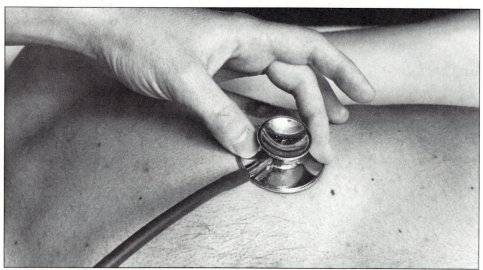

5 When you auscultate your patient, you use a stethoscope to assess the sounds produced by various arteries, organs, and tissues.

To properly assess high-frequency sounds—for example, breath sounds, and first and second heart sounds (S_1 and S_2)—use the diaphragm side of your stethoscope's chest piece. Make sure the diaphragm's entire surface is positioned firmly on your patient's skin.

☎ *Nursing tip:* You'll improve the diaphragm's contact and reduce extraneous noise by applying water or water-soluble jelly to your patient's chest before auscultating.

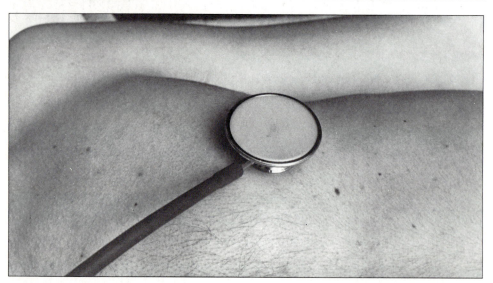

6 Suppose you want to use your stethoscope to assess low-frequency sounds; for example, heart murmurs, and third and fourth heart sounds (S_3 and S_4). *Lightly* place the stethoscope's bell on your patient's skin in the appropriate area. Never exert pressure on the bell. If you do, your patient's chest will act as a diaphragm, and you'll miss low-frequency sounds.

☎ *Nursing tip:* If your patient's extremely thin or emaciated, use a pediatric chest piece on your stethoscope. (For details on how to select a stethoscope properly, see page 77.)

How to document unusual skin conditions

As you assess your patient's skin, make sure you document the size, location, and extent of any skin abnormalities. Use a chart, such as the one illustrated here, to help. Here's how:

First, shade the body diagrams to match the locations of skin abnormalities on your patient's body. Number each area. Now, record those numbers, along with a complete, specific description of each abnormality, in the space provided below.

Attach the chart to your notes. Use it to determine if any *changes* occur in the patient's skin during your ongoing assessment.

How to assess your patient's pain

Since pain is a symptom of an underlying problem and (in many cases) is the complaint that brings a patient to a hospital, clinic, or doctor's office, learn how to identify and assess it properly.

As you know, your patient's reaction to pain depends on his individual personality and cultural environment. For example, he may not perceive pain as pain. Instead, he may refer to pain as an annoyance, an ache, a nuisance, or a discomfort. If so, be ready to substitute these words for pain during your patient interview.

Then, ask your patient the following questions, which cover six critical areas. Listen carefully to his answers, and document them.
- Location: *Where do you feel pain?*
- Quality: *Can you describe how the pain feels?*
- Quantity: *How intense is the pain?*
- Setting: *When did you first start having pain? Have you noticed any other problems or changes since it started?*
- Aggravating or alleviating factors: *What relieves the pain (if anything)? What makes it worse?*
- Associated signs and symptoms: *Do you notice any other problems or changes accompanying the pain?*

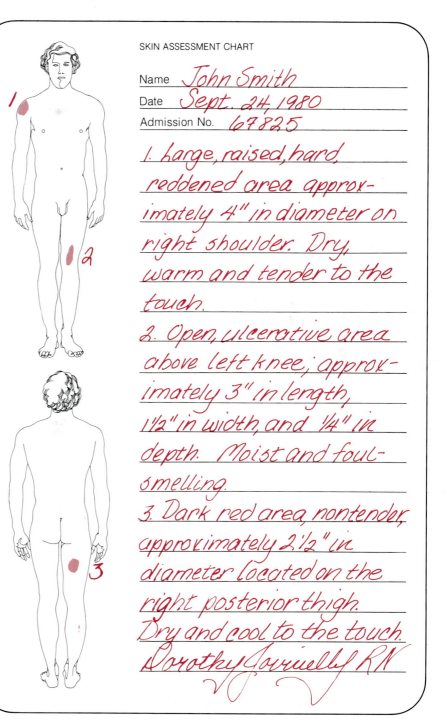

SKIN ASSESSMENT CHART

Name John Smith

Date Sept. 24, 1980

Admission No. 67825

1. Large, raised, hard, reddened area approximately 4" in diameter on right shoulder. Dry, warm and tender to the touch.

2. Open, ulcerative area above left knee; approximately 3" in length, 1½" in width, and ¼" in depth. Moist and foul-smelling.

3. Dark red area, nontender, approximately 2½" in diameter located on the right posterior thigh. Dry and cool to the touch.

Dorothy Gorinelly RN

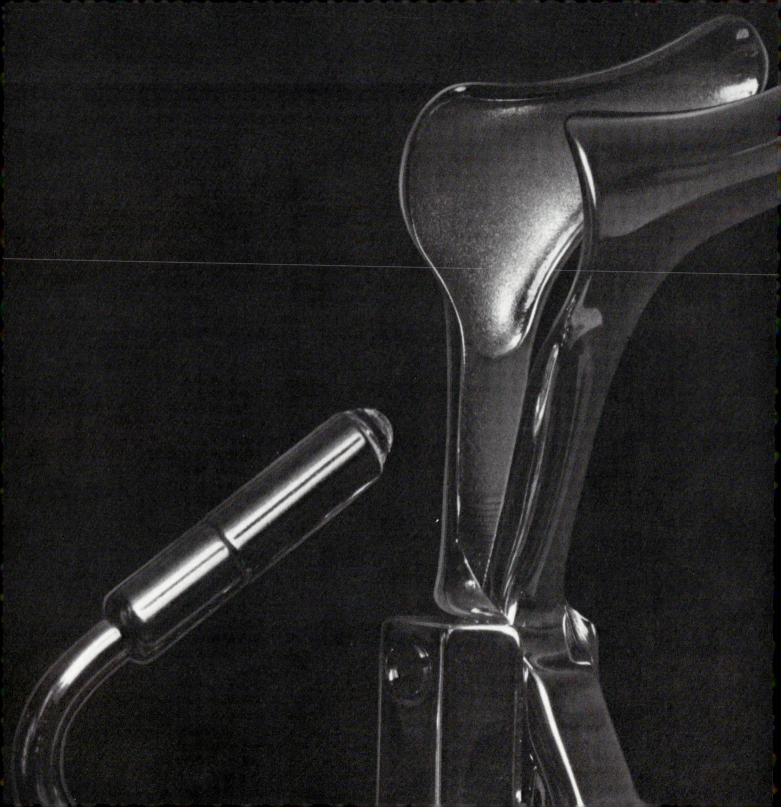

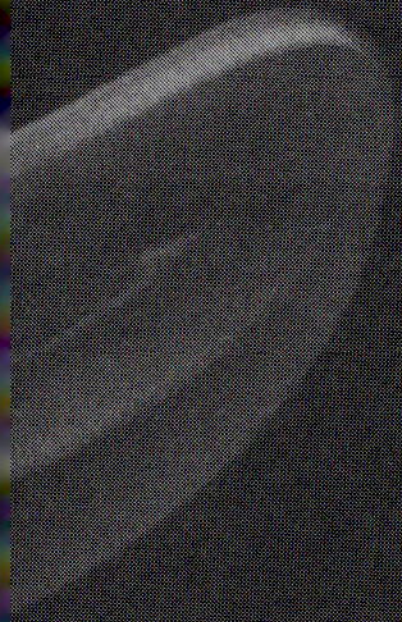

Examining the Head and Neck

Face, scalp, and neck inspection

Eye inspection

Ear inspection

Nose and sinus inspection

Mouth and throat inspection

Face, scalp, and neck inspection

What's the proper way to examine your patient's head and neck? Do you know what to look for? What signs may indicate an abnormality?

If you're not sure, study this section. On these pages, we'll:
• show you how to locate and assess your patient's lymph nodes.
• explain how to palpate his scalp.
• teach you how to test the range of motion in your patient's neck.

Remember, you can ease the anxiety your patient probably feels by explaining the examination and its purpose thoroughly before you begin.

DOCUMENTING

Head and neck questions: What to ask

Knowing how your patient perceives her health is an important part of your assessment. So before you begin examining her head and neck, ask questions that will help you zero in on her problems. The information you receive will serve as baseline data, so document it carefully.

Use the questions below as guidelines. Adjust or add to them to suit your patient's needs.
• Is your scalp itchy or flaking? Do you treat it with anything? Have you changed your shampoo recently?
• Do you have a hair loss problem? If so, is it generalized or in patches?
• Is there a history of baldness in your family?
• Have you had an injury or surgery on your head? If so, how long ago? Describe the details.
• Have you noticed any lumps or growths in your neck? Have you ever been treated for a goiter? Have you ever had surgery on your neck? If so, how long ago? Explain the reason.
• Have you ever had a tracheostomy? If so, how long ago? Explain the reason.
• Do you ever suffer from a stiff neck? If so, how often? How do you treat it?
• Do you have any other problems with your head or neck?

Locating your patient's lymph nodes, trachea, and thyroid gland

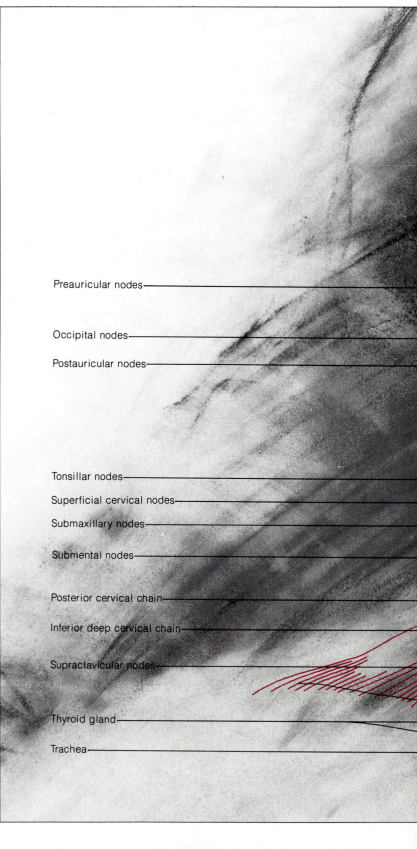

Preauricular nodes

Occipital nodes

Postauricular nodes

Tonsillar nodes

Superficial cervical nodes

Submaxillary nodes

Submental nodes

Posterior cervical chain

Inferior deep cervical chain

Supraclavicular nodes

Thyroid gland

Trachea

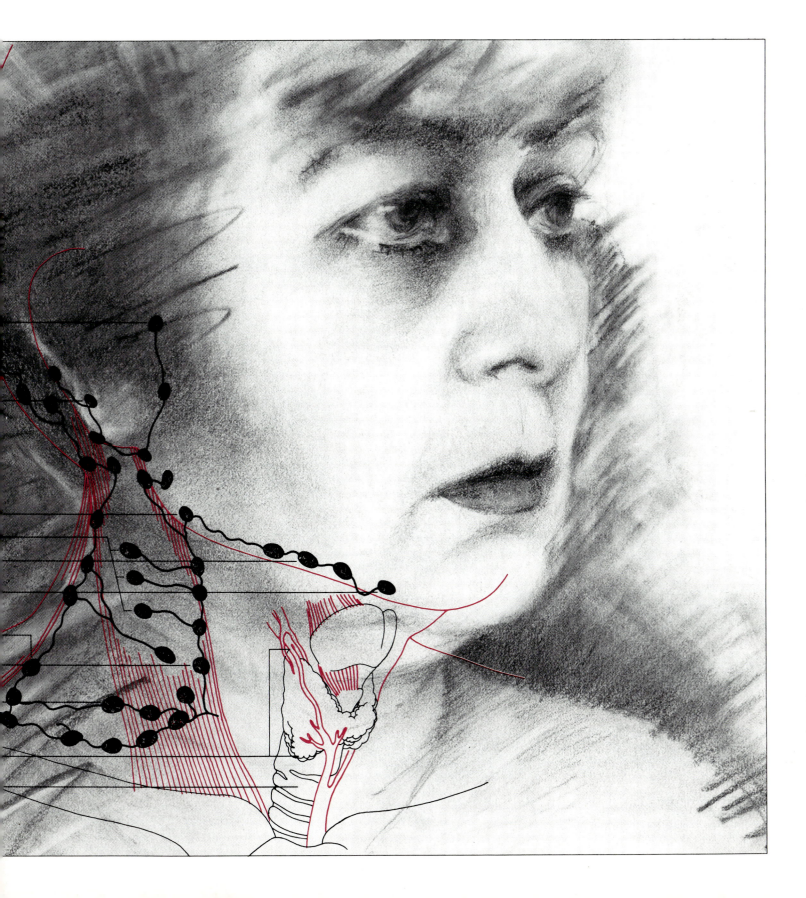

Face, scalp, and neck inspection

How to inspect your patient's head and neck

1 Begin your examination of your patient's head and neck by noting the size and contour of her skull. Observe the skin color of her face and neck. Then, check her scalp, face, and neck for lesions, scars, and involuntary movements.

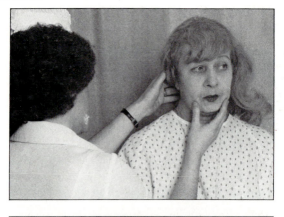 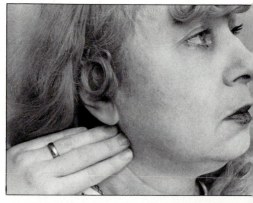

2 Now, gently palpate each temporal artery with your fingertips. If all's well, you'll feel a quick, steady pulse rate.

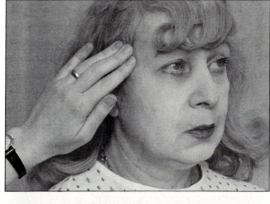 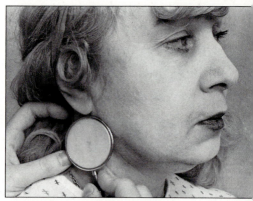

3 Next, inspect your patient's hair, and note its thickness, distribution, and texture. To visualize your patient's scalp, separate her hair into sections, with a wide-toothed comb. Palpate her scalp to look for possible tender areas, soft spots, bone movement, scales, lesions, cuts, and nits (lice eggs).

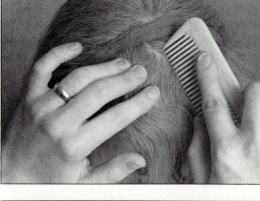 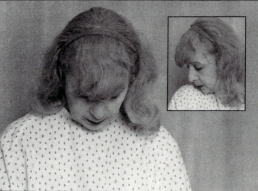

4 Now, observe your patient's neck. Check for asymmetry, abnormal pulsations, jugular vein distention, or an enlarged thyroid gland.

Assess her neck's range of motion. To test it, ask her to touch her chin to her chest, as shown here.

Then, ask her to touch her chin to her right shoulder (see inset).

Repeat the procedure, testing the left side of your patient's neck.

Does she have any difficulty with this range-of-motion exercise? If so, document it in your nurses' notes.

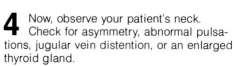 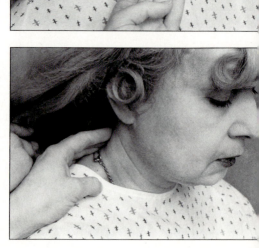

5 Locate your patient's right carotid artery, in the groove between her trachea and her sternocleidomastoid muscle. Gently palpate the artery to check the pulse rate and blood flow. Then, repeat this procedure on the patient's left side.

Important: Never apply pressure to a carotid artery. Doing so may cause your patient to develop bradycardia or asystole.

6 Use the stethoscope bell to auscultate your patient's right carotid artery for bruits (abnormal sounds caused by turbulent blood flow).

 Nursing tip: Ask your patient to hold her breath briefly while you auscultate her carotid artery. By doing this, you won't mistake air movement sounds for a bruit.

Repeat your auscultation on her left carotid artery.

7 Now, palpate your patient's lymph nodes. To do this, tip her head toward the area you'll be examining.

Now, using the illustration on pages 24 and 25 as a guide, locate your patient's right submental and submaxillary nodes. Also, locate the tonsillar node (see inset).

To do this, hook your fingers under her jaw. Place your fingertips directly over the area you'll be palpating. Then, palpate the nodes by sliding the skin back and forth over them. As you do, note their size, shape, mobility, hardness, and tenderness.

Repeat the procedure on her left side.

8 Next, ask your patient to tilt her head slightly forward. Locate her inferior deep cervical, posterior cervical, and supraclavicular nodes. To do this, hook your finger around her sternocleidomastoid muscle, as shown here. Palpate these nodes as before, checking for size, shape, mobility, hardness, and tenderness (if any).

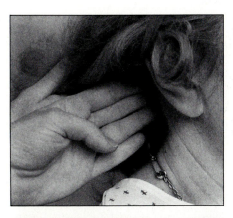

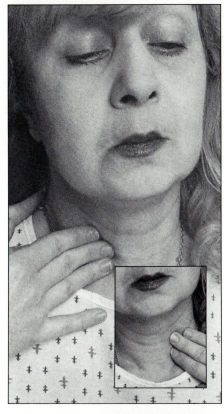

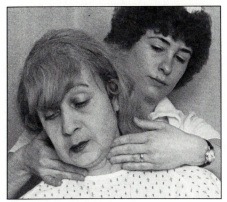

9 Now, locate and palpate your patient's right occipital node, as the nurse is doing in this photo. Then palpate her left occipital node.

Also, locate and palpate the preauricular and postauricular nodes. Note any abnormalities.

10 Palpate the patient's trachea. To do this, slip your fingertips into the sternal notch, and slide them to the right of the trachea.

[Inset] Then, slide them to the left side of the trachea. Check the trachea for possible deviations or displacement from the midline.

11 Now, move behind your patient. Ask her to tilt her head slightly forward and to the right. With your left hand, move her thyroid cartilage slightly to the right. Palpate her thyroid gland with your right hand. It should feel smooth, firm, and nontender. Tell your patient to swallow, to check for thyroid gland enlargement.

Repeat the procedure to check her other side.

Note: Is the thyroid gland enlarged? Use a stethoscope to check for bruits on either side of the isthmus—a sign of possible hyperthyroidism or severe endemic goiter.

Finally, document your findings.

Eye inspection

You may know something about eye examinations. But do you have the special knowledge and skills you'll need to accurately and thoroughly assess your patient's eyes?

For example, do you know:
* what findings indicate hypertension?
* how to test your patient for color blindness?
* how to select an ophthalmoscope aperture?
* how to test a patient's extraocular movement?

The following pages hold the answers to these questions, as well as many other important facts you'll want to know.

DOCUMENTING

Eye questions: What to ask

Always interview your patient carefully before you perform an eye examination. Why? Because questioning may prompt your patient to reveal signs and symptoms you should investigate. Do you know what questions to ask? If not, use this list as a guide. Ask your patient:

* How would you rate your vision? Excellent? Good? Fair? Or poor?
* Have you noticed any change in your vision lately? If so, describe the change.
* When was your last eye exam? Did you get a prescription for corrective lenses at that time? If so, do you need them for reading, for distance, or both? When did you get your last corrective lenses?
* Is your vision blurry? If so, when does the blurriness occur? Is the blurriness more frequent in the morning, afternoon, evening, or night?
* How would you rate your night vision?
* Have you ever had double vision? If so, describe the details.
* Do you ever see halos or colored rings around lights? If so, when?
* Do you have pain or discomfort in either eye? If so, describe it. Have you been treated for it? Does anything relieve it?
* Do you have discharge, crusting, or drainage from either eye? If so, can you describe it? What color is it? What consistency? Does it have an odor?
* Have you ever had an eye injury? If so, describe the details.
* Have you ever had eye surgery? If so, describe the details.
* Any other problems? For example, a history of diabetes or glaucoma?

As you interview your patient, observe her eyes separately and then compare them. Ask yourself these questions:
* Are your patient's eyes in line with the pinna of her ear?
* Is the sclera of each eye white, with a colored iris and a central dark pupil?
* Is there any redness, discharge, tearing, or swelling in either eye?
* When your patient's looking at you, is her gaze direct? Or do her eyes cross? Does either eye deviate upward or downward?

When you've completed these questions, be sure to document your findings in your notes.

Looking into the eye

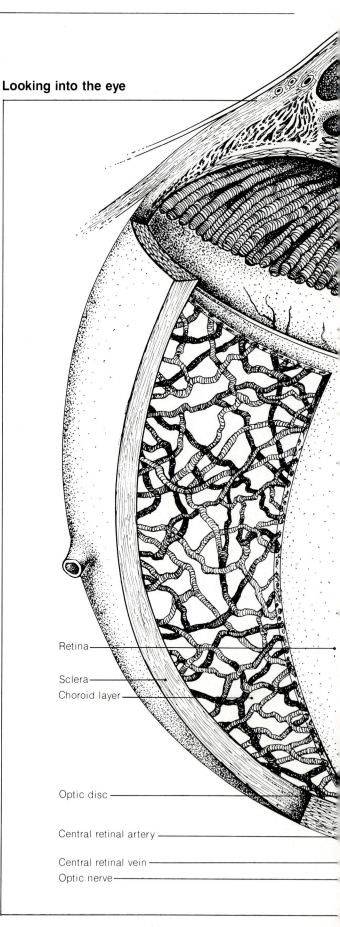

Retina

Sclera

Choroid layer

Optic disc

Central retinal artery

Central retinal vein

Optic nerve

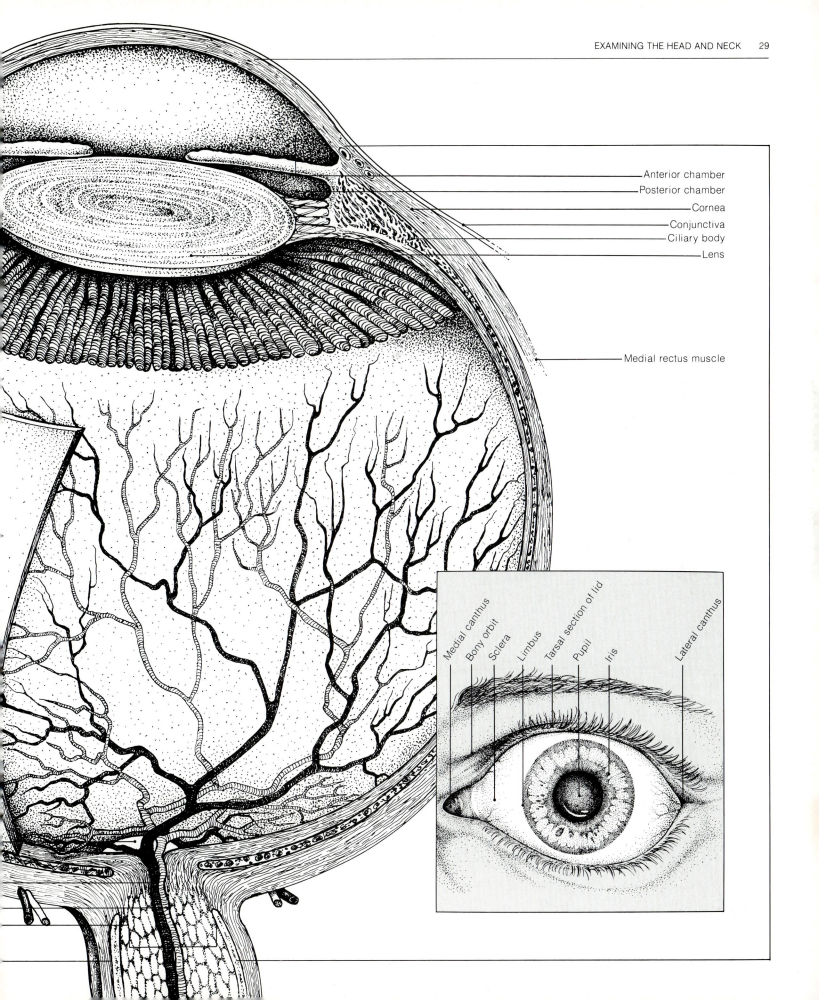

Anterior chamber
Posterior chamber
Cornea
Conjunctiva
Ciliary body
Lens

Medial rectus muscle

Medial canthus
Bony orbit
Sclera
Limbus
Tarsal section of lid
Pupil
Iris
Lateral canthus

Eye inspection

How to inspect your patient's eyes

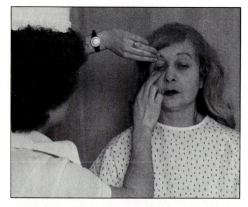

1 *Suppose you're examining your patient's eyes. Do you know what to look for? If not, study this photostory carefully.*

First, find a well-lighted, quiet area. Seat your patient so she's facing you. Then, palpate the orbital structure of her right eye, as shown in this photo. Look for lumps, bone movement, or tenderness.

Repeat the palpation on her left eye.

Important: Don't exert pressure on the eyeball. If you feel bone movement or your patient complains of pain, stop the examination immediately, and notify the doctor.

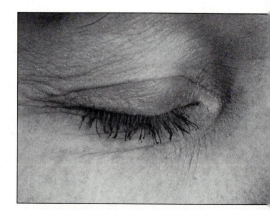

2 Next, ask your patient to close her eyes. Then, carefully palpate her right eye by gently sliding her eyelid over the eyeball, as shown here. On palpation, you'll notice that her eyeball yields slightly to pressure.

Repeat the procedure with her left eye.

If all's well, each eyeball will feel smooth and firm, and your patient will be able to identify touch sensation. If either eyeball feels soft and mushy or your patient complains of pain, stop the examination at once, and notify the doctor.

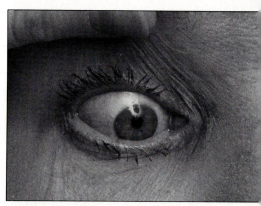

3 Now, ask your patient to open her eyes and focus on a point directly in front of her. If all's well, you'll notice both lower lid edges will meet at the bottom edges of the irises; and both upper lids will cover approximately 2 mm of the irises.

Suppose your patient's eyeballs protrude, causing her eyelids to retract. She may have a thyroid problem. Be sure to document your findings.

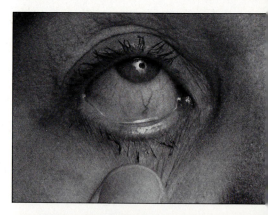

4 Next, ask your patient to open her eyes while you inspect the lash and lid edges of both eyes. If all's well, her lashes will be short, evenly spaced, and curl outward from both the upper and lower lids. Your patient's lid margins should appear pink and slightly moist. If you spot any abnormalities—for example, scales, crust, or discharge—document them.

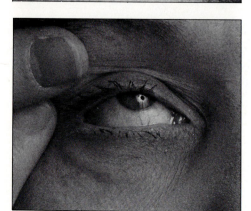

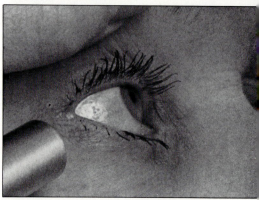

5 Observe how often your patient blinks. As you know, most people blink about 15 times a minute.

Now, instruct your patient to close her eyes. If everything's OK, her eyelids will meet, leaving no part of the sclerae, irises, or pupils visible. Note any abnormalities.

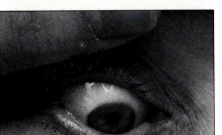

6 Ask your patient to open her eyes again, so you can examine the irises, pupils, and sclerae. Retract her upper right eyelid to observe her right iris. The iris will appear as a round, contoured disc centered in the sclera. Its radiating color lines should look even. If they look wavy, your patient may have had a lens removed.

As you look at your patient's iris, you'll see the pupil. Compare her right pupil to her left pupil. Note any differences in size or color, but keep in mind that some patients normally have unequal sized pupils.

Now check your patient's sclera.

7 To do this properly, you must also retract her lower eyelid. If all's well, the sclera will be white and moist. Note any growths, hemorrhages, or congested blood vessels.

Repeat the entire procedure on your patient's left eye.

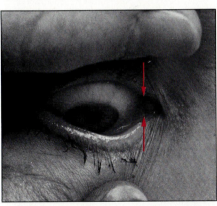

8 Next, inspect the right corneal surface. To do this, retract your patient's right upper lid. Then, shine a narrow beam of light at an angle across the corneal surface. If all's well, your patient's cornea will appear smooth, moist, and round. Note the size, texture, and clockface position of any opaque or cloudy areas in or near the cornea. Also, note any irregularities—for example, cuts or scratches—on the corneal surface.

If you notice any foreign bodies resting on or penetrating the surface, notify the doctor. Repeat your check on her left eye.

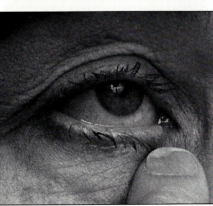

9 Now you'll examine the conjunctiva, which lines the back surface of your patient's eyelids. To do this, evert the right upper and lower lids, as explained on pages 32 and 33. If all's well, the conjunctiva will appear pink and clear. Note any inflammation, white or pale colorations, cuts, drainage, or cysts.

Repeat the procedure on your patient's left eye.

10 Now, ask your patient to look down and away from you. Using your thumb or index finger, slightly raise the upper lid of her right eye, noting any swelling of the lacrimal gland around the inner canthus.

11 Next, keeping the upper lid raised, retract your patient's lower lid, as shown here. You'll see the lacrimal puncta on the upper and lower lid margins, near the inner canthus (see arrows). Note any swelling, inflammation, or drainage.

12 Now, check the patency of the lacrimal duct. To do this, place your index finger on your patient's lower lid, below the lacrimal caruncle. Press gently. If you notice an excessive amount of discharge from the puncta, suspect an obstructed lacrimal duct.

Suppose you see pus in the discharged fluid. Suspect an infection.

Finally, palpate the lacrimal area, noting any extreme tenderness.

Repeat on your patient's left eye, and document your findings.

Eye inspection

How to evert an eyelid

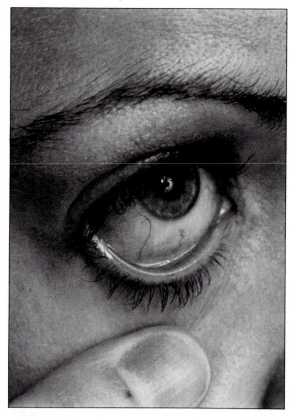

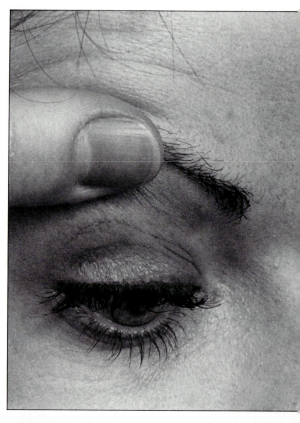

1 *To examine your patient's conjunctiva completely, you'll have to evert her eyelids. Can you do this safely and efficiently? If you're unsure, follow these guidelines:*

First, evert the lower lid, using your thumb or index finger. Gently retract the lid over the lower orbital rim.

2 Ask your patient to look up, then down, then left and right, as you examine her entire inner lid.

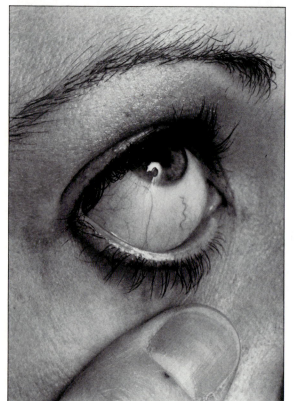

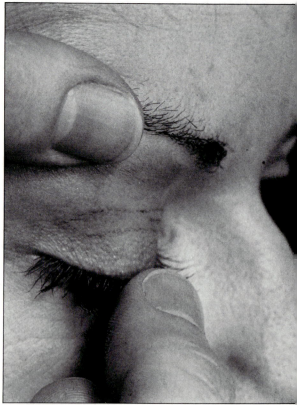

3 Now, ask your patient to look down while you evert her upper lid. To do this, slightly raise your patient's upper lid with your thumb or middle finger, as shown here. Take care not to press on her eyeball.

4 When her lashes protrude, gently grasp them between the thumb and index finger of your other hand.

5 Next, place the end of a cotton swab just above the eyelid fold.

6 Fold your patient's lid back over the cotton swab. With your fingers, secure the lid in this position. Remove the swab. Then, inspect the lid's inner lining, as shown here.

7 When your examination is completed, restore her upper lid to its normal position. To do this, ask your patient to look upward as you gently pull the lid forward.

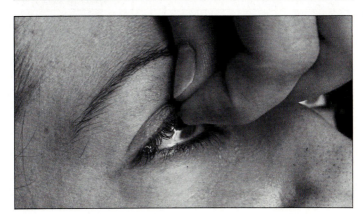

Eye inspection

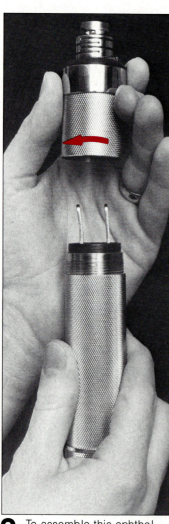

How to operate an ophthalmoscope

1 *As you know, an ophthalmoscope will help you identify possible inner eye abnormalities your patient may have. If you're unfamiliar with this assessment tool, study the assembly and operating guidelines in this photostory.*

In these photos, the nurse is using a Welch Allyn ophthalmoscope with a detachable battery pack. Along with the ophthalmoscope head, this model comes with an interchangeable otoscope, throat illuminator head, and nasal illuminator head.

2 To assemble this ophthalmoscope, screw the handle onto the battery housing, using a clockwise motion, as shown here.

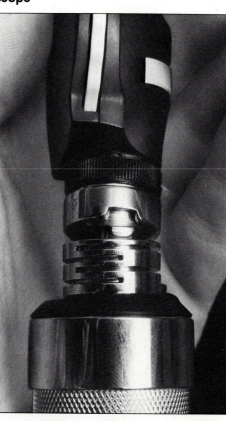

3 Next, align the slots in the base of the ophthalmoscope head with the lugs on the handle.

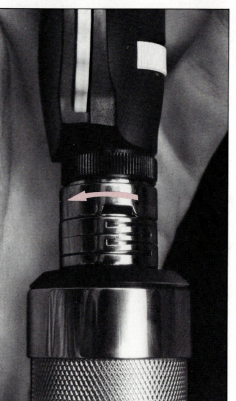

4 Firmly push the head down. Then, rotate it clockwise on the handle until you hear it click into place.

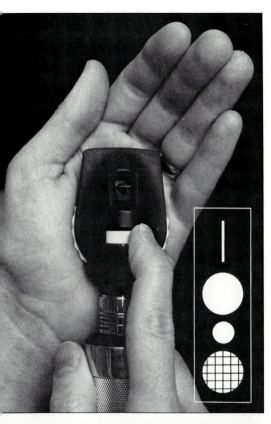

5 Now, locate the aperture selection dial on the back of the ophthalmoscope head, as shown here.

As you know, the aperture regulates the amount of light beamed into your patient's retina.

Rotate the aperture selection dial to choose the one that gives you the best visualization of your patient's eye. In most cases, you'll want to use the large, clear aperture.

[Inset] These illustrations show some of the other apertures you'll see as you rotate the aperture selection dial. If you're a trained professional, the grid and color apertures will help you make differential diagnoses on the eye.

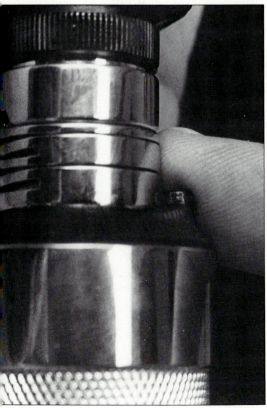

6 Now, get ready to select the correct aperture. Turn on the ophthalmoscope's light by pressing the red ON/OFF switch. Then, turn the black rheostat ring clockwise until it stops, as shown here. *Nursing tip:* To make aperture selection easy, hold the ophthalmoscope about 12" (30.5 cm) away from any flat surface; for example, a wall. Rotate the aperture selection dial until you see the correct aperture size reflected on the wall.

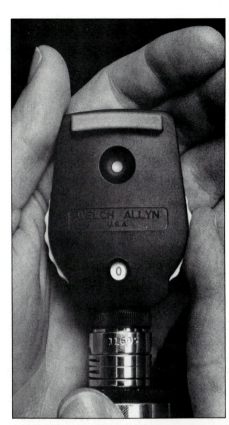

7 Choose the ophthalmoscope lens that best brings your patient's inner eye structure into focus. To do this, turn the ophthalmoscope head toward you, as shown.

Rotate the white dial (or lens selection disc) until you find a lens that brings the inner eye into focus.

Now, look for the illuminated lens indicator, below the lens opening. As you know, the numbers that appear in this indicator correspond to the selected lens's plus or minus sphere power.

If your patient's vision is normal, you've probably selected the 0, or neutral, lens. *Important:* Always note the lens power you use for your patient's examination.

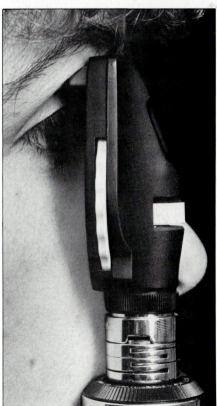

8 Finally, to hold the ophthalmoscope correctly, place the brow rest under your eyebrow, and look through the aperture, as shown here. Then, rest your index finger on the lens selection disc.

Remember: When you use the ophthalmoscope, always keep both eyes open to maintain your depth perception.

Eye inspection

Examining the eye with an ophthalmoscope

1 *You discovered how to assemble and operate an ophthalmoscope, on pages 34 and 35. Here's how to use it to examine your patient's eyes.*

First, seat your patient in a room that you can darken partially or completely. As you know, a darkened room will cause your patient's pupils to dilate, exposing more of her peripheral retina.

☎ *Nursing tip:* Place a lamp near your patient's chair, so *you'll* be able to see after the room's darkened.

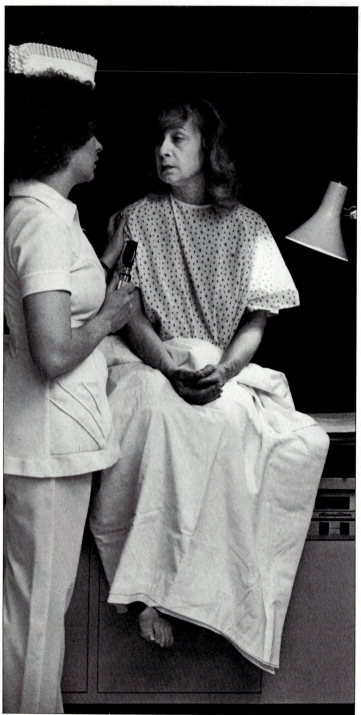

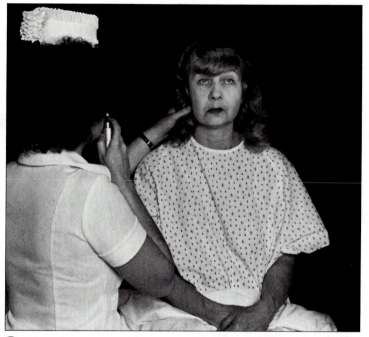

2 Now, darken the room. Sit or stand facing your patient at her eye level.

To examine your patient's right eye, position yourself on her right side, as shown here.

Hold the ophthalmoscope up to your right eye with your right hand, and illuminate it. Set the ophthalmoscope lens at 0 (unless contraindicated, as explained on page 35).

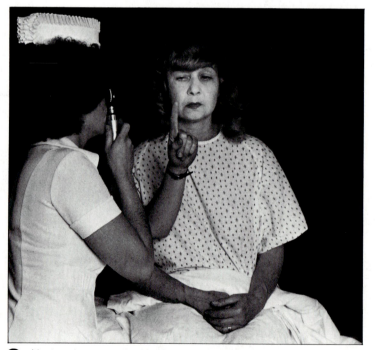

3 Next, ask your patient to focus on a stationary object at eye level. Hold the ophthalmoscope about 12" (30 cm) in front of her, and direct the beam of light at your patient's right pupil.

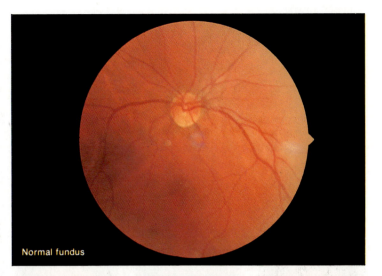

Normal fundus

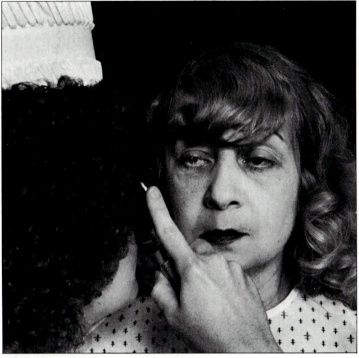

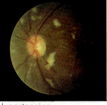
Glaucoma

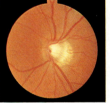
Hypertension

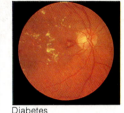
Diabetes

4 Slowly move the ophthalmoscope closer to your patient until you're about 6" (15.2 cm) from her right eye, as shown here. *Note:* You should be at a 25° angle to her right side.

[Inset, at left] Looking through the lens aperture, you'll see an orange glow, known as the red reflex, on her pupil. If you don't see the red reflex, your patient may have corneal lesions or a complete retinal detachment. Notify the doctor.

6 Get ready to examine the fundus. Study the top photo of a normal fundus so you know what to look for.

Begin by observing the color, clarity of the optic disc's outline, and the elevation and condition of the blood vessels.

If the optic disc appears enlarged and gray (with white edges), your patient may have glaucoma. Recommend that she see a trained professional to have her intraocular pressure measured.

Suppose the optic disc's obscured and you see flame-shaped hemorrhages (some near disc edges), and tufts of exudate. Your patient may have hypertension. Notify the doctor.

Now, locate the macula, which is about 3 mm from the optic disc's temporal edge. The macula, which normally has no blood vessels, should appear darker than the surrounding areas.

Suppose the macula is spotted with white exudate and the retinal edges have irregular vessels, with small aneurysms, hemorrhages, and patches of white exudate. Your patient may have diabetes. Notify the doctor.

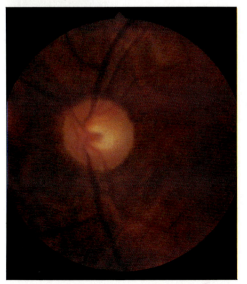

5 Now, move the ophthalmoscope toward your patient's eye until you visualize the optic disc. If all's well, the optic disc will be yellowish, and round or oval in shape.

Look for the optic disc cup, which is a white, central depression one third the size of the disc. As you probably know, the nasal edge of the cup will be less distinct than the temporal edge. You may also see a white crescent around the temporal edge.

Suppose the optic disc appears out of focus. Rotate the lens selection disc (white dial) until you can clearly visualize the disc.

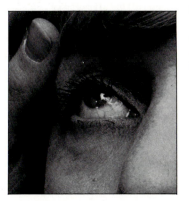

7 Next, inspect the peripheral areas of the fundus. To do this, instruct your patient to look up, then to one side, and then toward her nose. Note any capillary hemorrhages, white patches, opacities, or dilated vessels.

Repeat the entire examination on your patient's left eye.

Eye inspection

How to test color blindness

Planning to test your patient's color vision? You'll need a set of pseudoisochromatic or polychromatic plates and a well-lighted area.

Important: The illustrations shown here are simply an artist's *interpretation* of the type of plates you'll use to test your patient's color blindness. *They are not color reproductions of actual plates and must not be used for testing.*

As you can see from these illustrations, a pseudoisochromatic or polychromatic plate is composed of an arrangement of colored dots. Within the arrangement, similar colors make up a number, letter, or shape on a contrasting background.

To test your patient's color vision, first ask her if she's noticed any problems identifying colors. Then, hold the plates at arm's length (30" to 40" or 75 to 100 cm) in front of her. *Note:* Never test your patient with the plates closer than arm's length. If you do, the test results will be inaccurate.

Now, instruct your patient to study each plate for 3 to 5 seconds only, as you page through the book. Note any difficulty she may have distinguishing the number, letter, or shape on each plate.

Suppose your patient is a child or illiterate. Ask your patient to *trace* the path she sees within the plate.

To determine what's considered normal, consult the score sheet or chart included with your set of plates. It'll describe what a patient with normal color vision sees and what a patient with a color deficiency (of any type) sees.

As you know, color blindness varies in type and severity. Red-green color blindness is the most common. Blue-yellow and total color blindness are rare. Because some plates are designed only to detect red-green color blindness, a person with blue-yellow color blindness will pass the test successfully. Study the instructions with your set of plates carefully before testing your patient's color vision.

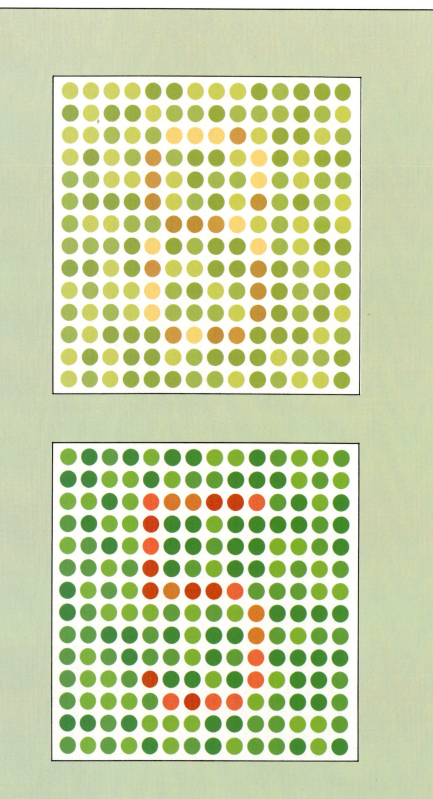

How to test extraocular movement

1 *Suppose you're testing your patient's extraocular movement. Begin by familiarizing yourself with the six cardinal fields of gaze shown in this photo.* As you know, each of these fields corresponds to one of your patient's extraocular muscles. Check each field separately, as explained below.

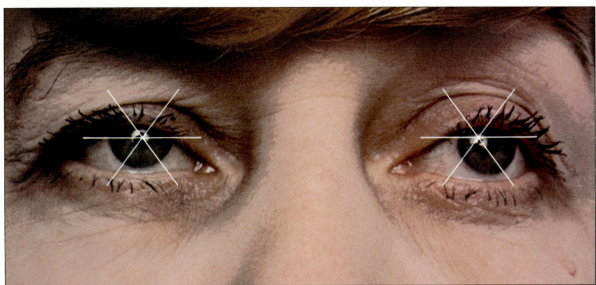

2 First, hold a pencil 12" (30 cm) in front of your patient's nose.

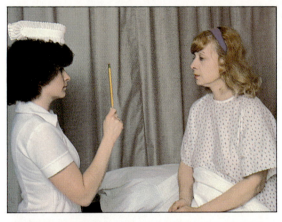

3 Ask her to hold her head still and to follow the pencil's movement with her eyes. Then, slowly move the pencil to your patient's right side, as shown here. Observe both her eyes simultaneously. When the pencil's approximately 2' (60 cm) from your starting point, or your patient's eye movement stops (in either or both eyes), hold the pencil still. Note the position of the iris in relation to each eye's midline.

Repeat this procedure, checking each vision field separately.

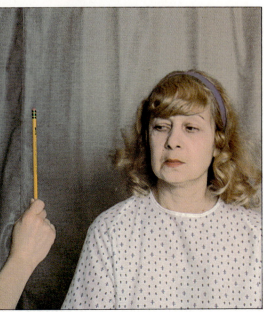

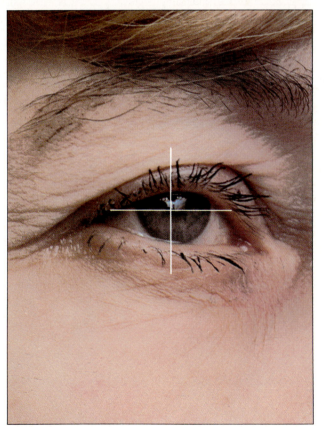

4 How do you evaluate the results? Picture your patient's eyeball as a grid divided into quarters.

If her extraocular movements are within normal ranges, your patient will be able to move each eye so the edge of the iris approaches the grid's center. Stay alert for abnormal eye movement; for example, jerking, oscillation, eyes not tracking together, or lagging lids. These signs indicate possible extraocular muscle problems.

Eye inspection

How to test accommodation and convergence

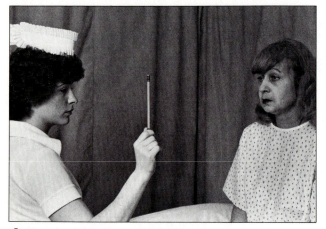

1 *If you're testing your patient's accommodation and convergence, follow these steps:*
First, hold a pencil approximately 18" (45.7 cm) in front of your patient's nose. Then, ask her to watch the pencil as you move it. Instruct her to keep her head and eyes stationary throughout the exam.

2 Slowly move the pencil toward the bridge of her nose. If everything's OK, both your patient's eyes will converge on the pencil at the same level and distance. At that point, expect her pupils to constrict and remain constricted.
When the pencil's 2" to 3" (5 to 7.6 cm) from the bridge of her nose, your patient should be able to comfortably hold her gaze.
Document all findings in your nurses' notes.

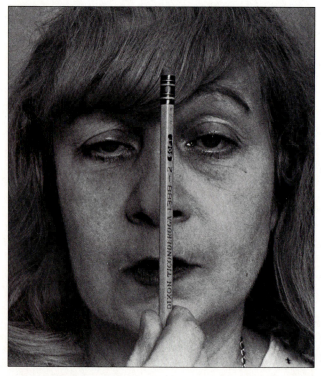

How to test visual acuity

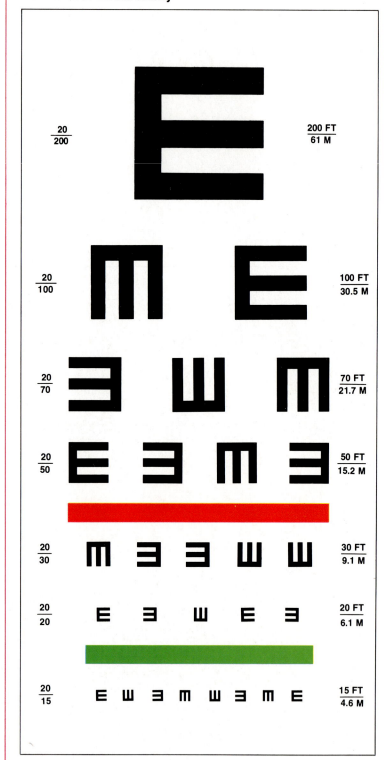

20/200	200 FT / 61 M
20/100	100 FT / 30.5 M
20/70	70 FT / 21.7 M
20/50	50 FT / 15.2 M
20/30	30 FT / 9.1 M
20/20	20 FT / 6.1 M
20/15	15 FT / 4.6 M

1 *Testing your patient's visual acuity? You'll need a Snellen chart or an E chart, like the one shown here.*
🔖 *Nursing tip:* To avoid embarrassing your patient, always ask if she can read English before you begin the examination. If she can't, use an E chart, or a picture chart.

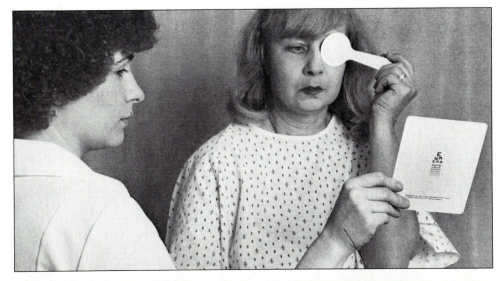

2 Begin by asking your patient to cover her left eye with a clean opaque card or occluder.

Then, if you're using a hand-held chart, hold the chart at your patient's eye level. Follow the manufacturer's instructions for recommended distance.

Suppose you're using a wall-mounted chart. Ask your patient to sit or stand at eye level 20' (6 m) from the chart.

Instruct your patient to read the smallest line on the chart she can see clearly. If her vision is normal, she'll be able to read the line marked *20/20*.

Document your findings.

3 Suppose your patient can't read the *20/20* line. Note the smallest line she can read with each eye, and record the number that corresponds to it.

What if your patient has difficulty reading even the largest letter on the chart? Move the chart closer to her (or move her closer to the chart), until she can see the largest letter clearly. Then, document the distance she was from the chart, and write that number over the number *200*. For example, if your patient was 10' (3 m) from the chart before she could read it, you'd record *10/200*.

4 Your patient may have difficulty reading the eye chart at any distance. If she does, test her visual acuity with a low-vision chart, as the nurse is doing here. Then, document your findings.

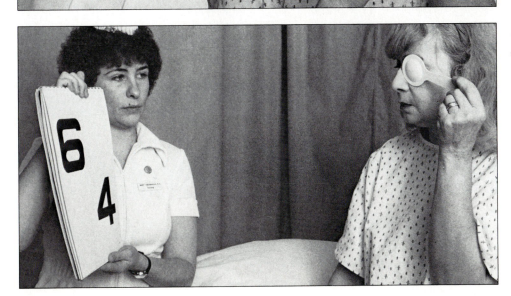

Eye inspection

Testing your patient's vision fields

1 *Suppose you're testing your patient's vision fields. Do you know how to proceed? If you're unsure, follow these steps:*

Begin by seating your patient on a chair or exam table in a well-lighted area. Then, sit or stand facing her, about 2' (61 cm) away. Make sure you and your patient are at eye level.

Important: Do you have an uncorrected vision problem? Don't attempt to test your patient's vision fields. Instead, ask someone else to do it.

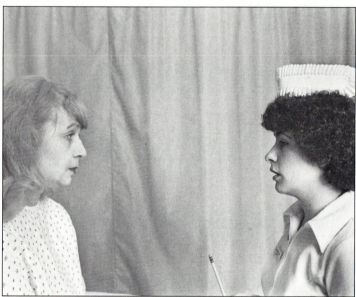

3 Now, hold a test object, such as a finger, penlight, or pencil, at arm's length above your head. Make sure the pencil is midway between you and your patient.

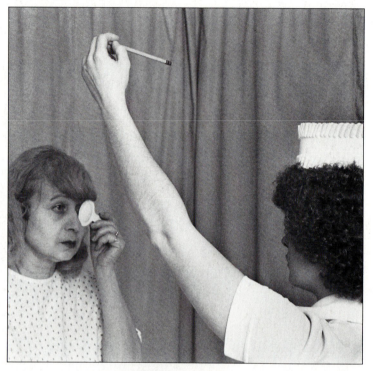

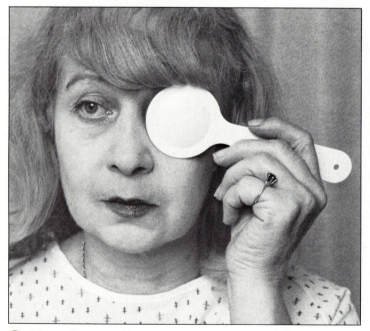

2 Now, tell your patient to close her left eye, as you close your *right* eye.

🔖 *Nursing tip:* If your patient can't close one eye, instruct her to cover the eye with a clean opaque card or occluder.

Next, look directly into each other's open eye. Instruct your patient to keep her head and eyes stationary during the examination.

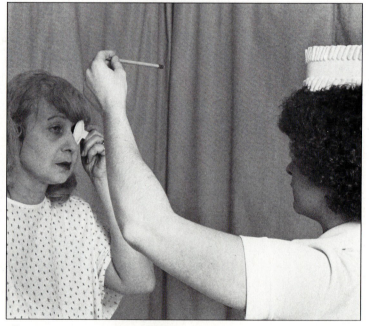

4 Slowly lower the pencil. Ask your patient to tell you when she first sees the pencil.

Compare the point where *she* sees the pencil to the point where *you* see the pencil. Note any differences.

Repeat the test with your patient's right eye closed and her left eye open. Then, keep *your* left eye closed and *your* right eye open.

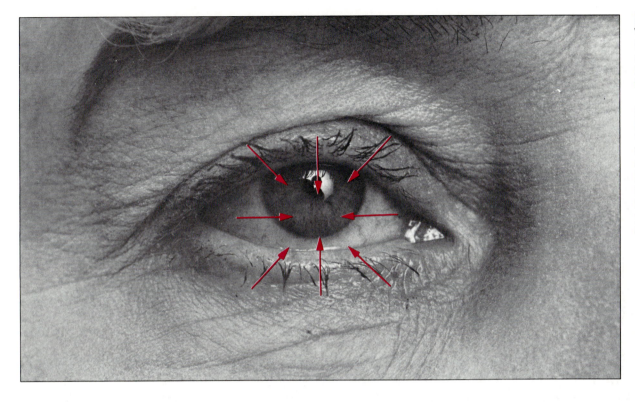

5 Now, repeat the same test for each of the eight directions shown by the arrows in this illustration.

Remember, if you're testing your patient's temporal vision field, start with the pencil slightly behind her. But keep in mind that this will bring the pencil into your line of vision *first*.

Recognizing common eye problems

Assessment variables	Acute conjunctivitis	Acute keratitis	Cataract	Acute narrow angle glaucoma	Detached retina
Discharge	• Watery to purulent	• Watery to purulent, or none	• None	• None	• None
Pain	• None	• Mild to severe	• None	• Severe	• None
Vision	• Normal	• Blurred	• Progressive blurring	• Blurred or sudden vision loss	• Part of vision field lost
Redness	• Generalized	• Redness more prominent at corneal-scleral margin	• None	• Redness more prominent at corneal-scleral margin	• None
Ophthalmoscopic exam	• Normal	• Interruption of red reflex may occur from corneal opacity.	• Lens may appear cloudy. • Retina may be difficult to see because of corneal opacity.	• Optic disc cup may be enlarged (usually greater than 1:2).	• Portion of retina may be seen suspended in the vitreous humor. • Cloudy vitreous humor. • Retinal tears look orange or red and appear crescent-shaped. • No red reflex
Pupillary changes	• None	• None	• Pupil appears white as cataract matures.	• Pupil moderately dilated. • Pupil won't react to light.	• None
Special	• Patient may complain of gritty sensation or burning in his eyes.	• When stain is applied to cornea, epithelial defect may be seen.	• None	• Intraocular pressure is elevated. • Halos around lights.	• In early stages, before vision loss, patient may see floating spots or flashes of light.

Ear inspection

How skilled are you at examining your patient's ears? For example, do you know how to recognize a patient with a conductive hearing loss? How to test hearing acuity with a tuning fork? How to interpret Weber, Rinne, or Schwabach test results? How to use an otoscope?

As you know, your ability to perform a complete and efficient ear examination will help you accurately assess your patient.

Review the following pages carefully. We've included charts, and photostories to help you sharpen your present assessment skills.

DOCUMENTING

Ear questions: What to ask

You'll need to know baseline information about your patient and her environment to conduct a thorough ear exam and hearing test. Here are some sample questions you may want to ask:

• How would you describe your hearing? Excellent? Good? Fair? Or poor?
• Have you ever had your hearing tested? If so, when? What were the results?
• Do you have any problems with either ear? What kind? Have you received any treatment for these problems?
• How do you feel when many people talk at the same time?
• Do you ever feel like you're missing parts of a conversation?
• Have you ever worked around noisy equipment? If so, when? For how long? Did you wear hearing protection?
• Do you ever hunt, or shoot at a rifle range? If so, what do you wear to protect your hearing? Do you shoot left- or right-handed?
• Have you noticed a change in your hearing? What kind? When did it occur?

• Do you ever have earaches? If so, how frequently? Did a doctor give you any medication for it? If so, do you know what kind?
• Have you had any ear injuries, infection, or surgery? If so, describe the details.
• Have you ever had any ear drainage or crusting in either ear? If so, which ear? Describe the color and odor.
• Do you ever have a full feeling in either ear? When?
• Do you ever feel dizzy? When? How long does it last?
• Any other problems?

While you ask your patient these questions, make your own observations. Ask yourself these questions:
• Is my patient tilting her head toward me when I speak?
• Has my patient asked me to repeat any questions? Are her answers appropriate?
• Is there any discharge or crusting in either ear?
• Does my patient have any obvious malformation or deficiencies in either ear?

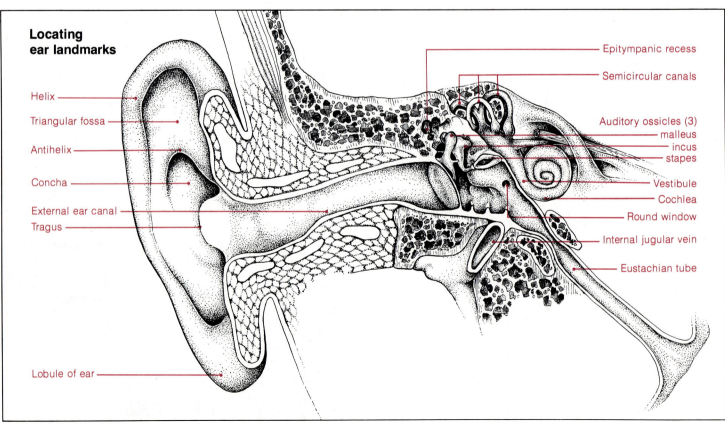

Locating ear landmarks

Helix

Triangular fossa

Antihelix

Concha

External ear canal

Tragus

Lobule of ear

Epitympanic recess

Semicircular canals

Auditory ossicles (3)
malleus
incus
stapes

Vestibule

Cochlea

Round window

Internal jugular vein

Eustachian tube

Assembling and operating the otoscope

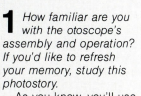

1 *How familiar are you with the otoscope's assembly and operation? If you'd like to refresh your memory, study this photostory.*

As you know, you'll use the same battery housing and handle for the otoscope that you use for the ophthalmoscope. (For details on this, see page 34.)

This photo shows an otoscope head, which includes a light source and magnifying lens, and various sized specula attachments.

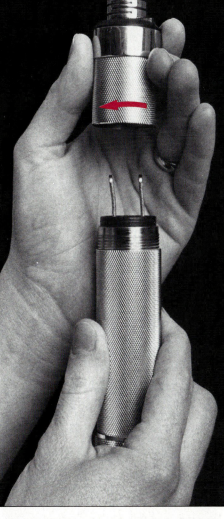

2 Are you using a model that you can recharge in a wall unit? If you are, attach the battery pack to the handle, as shown here. Then screw the handle onto the battery housing, using a clockwise motion.

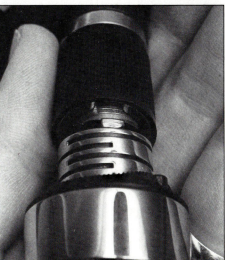

3 Now, attach the otoscope head. To do this, hold the handle in one hand and the head in your other hand (with the lugged side down).

Ear inspection

Assembling and operating the otoscope continued

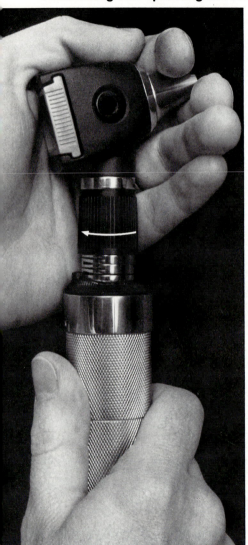

4 Now, align the lugs on the otoscope head with the notches on the handle. Push the head down firmly. Then, twist the head in a clockwise direction, until it clicks into place.

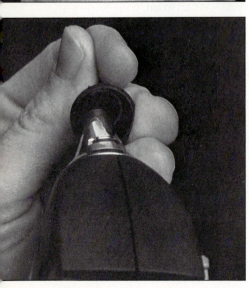

5 Next, attach an ear speculum—the largest one comfortable for your patient. To do this, use your free hand to align the speculum's inside notch with the notch on the otoscope head. Gently snap the speculum into the otoscope head, and secure it.

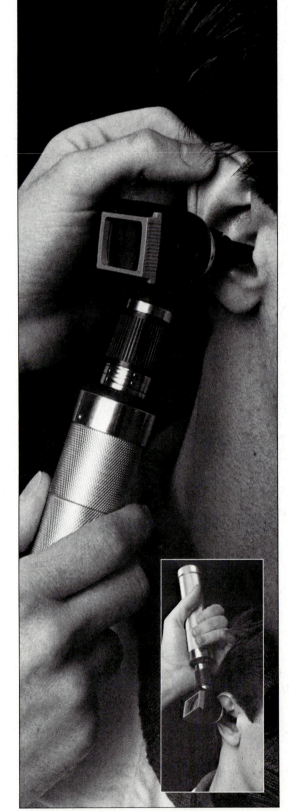

6 Now, to properly examine your patient's ear, hold the otoscope handle down, as shown here.

[Inset] Suppose your patient's uncooperative; for example, a frightened child. Hold the otoscope handle up, with the side of your hand resting against the side of your patient's head. Doing so will help you brace the otoscope and prevent ear damage if your patient moves.

Important: If you're using an otoscope other than the model we've featured in these photos, follow the manufacturer's assembly and operation instructions.

Examining the ear

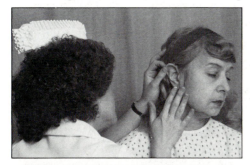

1 *If you're performing an ear examination on your patient, you'll need an otoscope and several different sized ear specula.*

Explain the procedure to your patient, and reassure her. Then, follow these instructions to perform the examination:

First, tilt your patient's head slightly away from you, so you can see her ear clearly. Then, inspect her external ear canal, noting any abnormalities, such as discharge, skin lesions, or lumps. If you see any foreign bodies in the ear canal, notify the doctor.

2 If you see any discharge or your patient complains of pain, check for tenderness by gently moving the auricle with your fingers, as shown in this photo.

[Inset] Also press the tragus and mastoid process. If your patient complains of pain, she may have otitis externa or mastoiditis.

3 Now, straighten the ear canal as much as possible. To do this for an adult, pull the auricle upward and backward.

4 With your patient's ear canal properly positioned, begin examining her internal ear canal with an otoscope. Select the largest speculum that fits comfortably in your patient's ear.

Nursing tip: If your patient is restless or unable to sit up for an exam, position her on her side on a bed or exam table. But make sure the ear you're examining is facing up.

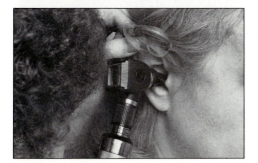

5 Now, *gently* insert the speculum tip slightly forward and downward into your patient's ear canal. But never force it. If you meet resistance, the speculum's probably too large. Replace it.

If you still meet resistance, notify the doctor.

Ear inspection

Examining the ear continued

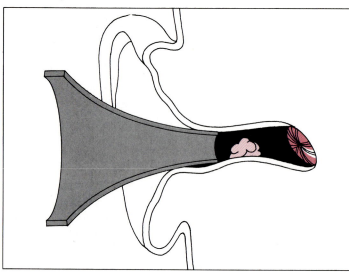

6 Now, look through the otoscope for the patient's eardrum. To do this, gently advance the speculum a little way into the ear canal. Expect to see a little brown or orange wax (cerumen) along the smooth pink walls.

Note: If a large wax plug partially or completely occludes your view, remove the speculum and notify the doctor. He may order an ear irrigation to remove the plug. (For information on how to irrigate a patient's ear, see the NURSING PHOTOBOOKS *Dealing with Emergencies* or *Giving Medications.*)

Always document any redness, swelling, lesions, or scales you see along the ear canal. Also keep in mind that this procedure will be painful if your patient's ear is inflamed.

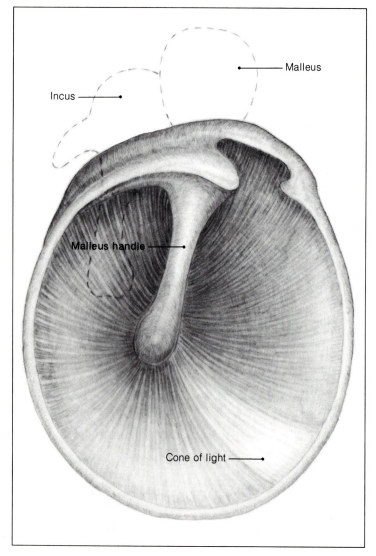

Incus

Malleus

Malleus handle

Cone of light

7 When you see the eardrum, carefully angle the speculum for the best view. If everything's OK, the eardrum will look like a shiny pearl-gray or pale pink disc that's slightly coned inward. However, a deep pink or red eardrum may indicate inflammation; a bulging, white eardrum may indicate drainage in the middle ear; and a blue eardrum may indicate accumulated blood.

Behind the eardrum you'll see the malleus handle, which extends downward in the center of the eardrum.

If the eardrum's properly positioned, look for a cone of light at the 5-o'clock position in the right ear, and at the 7-o'clock position in the left ear.

If the cone of light is displaced or absent, your patient's eardrum may be bulging, retracted, or inflamed.

Document your findings.

How to test your patient's gross hearing

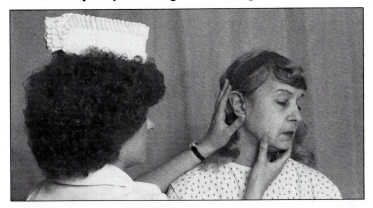

1 *Wondering how to evaluate your patient's hearing? First, test her gross hearing using the voice and the watch-tick tests.*

Select a quiet room or area to conduct your testing. Then, explain the testing routine to your patient, and seat her on a chair or an exam table. Make sure her right ear's in front of you.

Remember: Before you begin any hearing test, check your patient's ear for cerumen accumulation. Ask if she has a cold. As you know, either of these conditions may interfere with your patient's hearing ability.

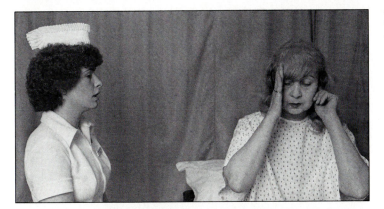

2 Now, ask your patient to mask the hearing in her left ear by placing her left index fingertip into her left external ear canal. Instruct her to rapidly move her fingertip in and out of the canal, as shown here.

[Inset] If your patient has long fingernails, tell her to block the ear opening with the tragus.

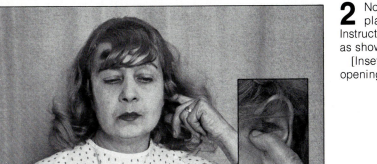

3 Now, position yourself about 2' (61 cm) from your patient. Then, so she won't be able to read your lips, ask her to block her vision by holding her right hand to the right side of her face, as shown here. Or if you have an opaque card or a file folder, ask her to hold it against the side of her face.

Next, whisper any three of these words toward your patient's right ear: *three, nine, bell, later, kill, light,* or *might.*

If all's well, your patient will be able to repeat all three words. If she can't, say them again in a loud whisper. If she still can't repeat the words, speak them aloud.

Now, test your patient's left ear. But remember, choose three different words, so your patient won't rely on her memory to repeat the words.

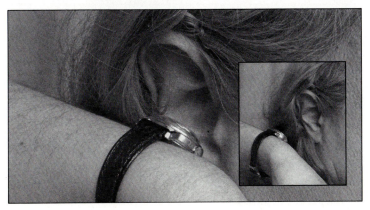

4 Instruct your patient to maintain the same position while you perform the watch-tick test.

As before, ask her to mask the hearing in her left ear with her fingertip. Then, place a watch face directly in front of your patient's right ear, as the nurse is doing here. Ask your patient if she hears the ticking.

[Inset] If she hears the ticking, gradually move the watch away from her ear. Note how far away it is when your patient can no longer hear the ticking.

If all's well, your patient will hear the ticking a maximum of 4" to 6" (10 to 15 cm) from each ear.

Now, while she masks the hearing in her right ear, use the same watch to test the hearing in her left ear.

Finally, document the test results in your nurses' notes.

Ear inspection

How to test your patient's hearing acuity

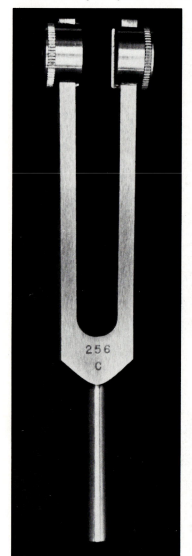

1 *Testing your patient's hearing acuity? If so, you'll need a tuning fork in the C octave. In this photostory, we're using a 256-hertz tuning fork to perform the Weber, Rinne, or Schwabach tests.*

By studying the results of these tests, a trained health-care professional can differentiate between a patient with normal hearing and a patient with a conductive or sensorineural hearing loss.

To ensure accurate results, you should perform each of these tests three separate times with 256-, 512-, and 1,024-hertz tuning forks. However, this may not always be possible.

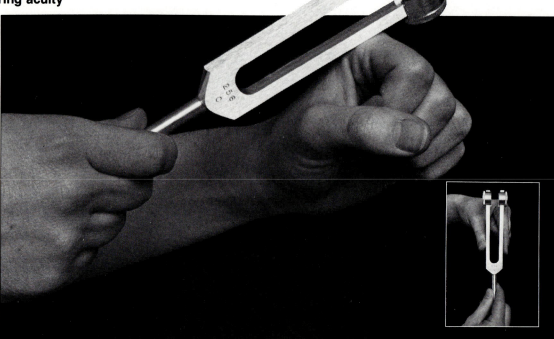

2 Before you begin a test, explain the testing procedure to your patient. Then, practice vibrating the tuning fork.

You'll get the most accurate testing tone by gently hitting the fork against your fist.

[Inset] You may also get a tone by pinching the fork's prongs together, or by stroking the prongs upward.

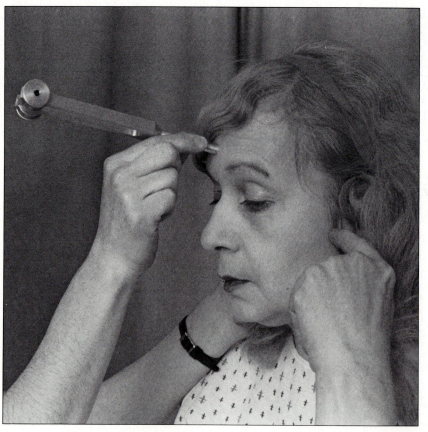

3 Now you're ready to perform the Weber test. Begin by holding a *vibrating* 256-hertz tuning fork between your thumb and index finger. Touch the base of the tuning fork to your patient's forehead.

Then, ask your patient to describe the tone in each ear. If all's well, your patient will hear the same tone (volume and intensity) in each ear. In that case, you'd document the result as *Weber negative.*

If your patient hears the tone louder in one ear, ask her to point to the ear in which she hears the louder tone. Document the result *Weber right* or *Weber left.*

4 Next, you'll perform the Rinne test to evaluate your patient's hearing by both bone and air conduction. Here's how:

First, ask your patient to mask the hearing in her left ear by rapidly moving her left fingertip in and out of her left ear canal.

To test your patient's hearing by bone conduction, place the vibrating 256-hertz fork against her right mastoid process. Your patient should hear the tone immediately. Ask her to tell you when she no longer hears the tone. Note the length of time she heard the tone.

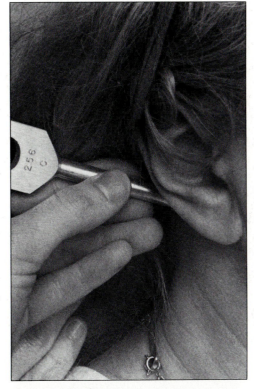

6 Now, you'll perform the Schwabach test to compare *your* hearing by bone conduction with *your patient's* hearing by bone conduction. But remember, make sure your hearing is normal before you begin or the test won't be accurate.

Ask your patient to mask the sound in her left ear, as explained before. Then, place a vibrating 256-hertz tuning fork on her right mastoid process until she says she hears the sound. If all's well, she should say she hears the sound immediately.

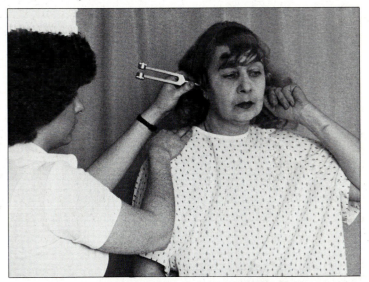

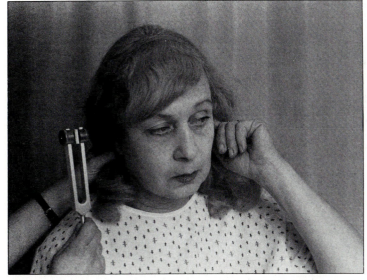

5 Then, test her hearing by air conduction. Quickly (without revibrating the fork), place the prongs ½" (1.3 cm) from her right external ear canal, as the nurse is doing here. Make sure the prongs are in front of—but not touching—the ear canal.

Ask your patient to tell you when she no longer hears the tone. Note the length of time she heard the tone. If everything's OK, your patient will hear the tone carried by air conduction twice as long as the tone carried by bone conduction.

In this case, document the results as +R (Rinne positive). (See the chart on page 52 for information on how to document other results.)

Repeat the same procedure on your patient's left ear.

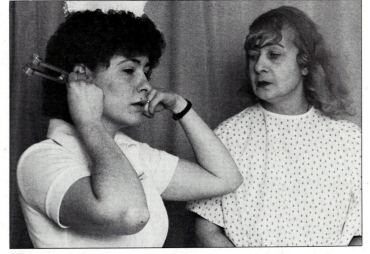

7 Then, immediately mask the sound in *your* left ear, and place the fork on *your* right mastoid process. Listen for the sound.

Continue to alternate the tuning fork between your patient's mastoid process and your mastoid process. When either you or your patient stops hearing the tone, count the seconds the other continues to hear it.

If both of you have normal hearing, you'll stop hearing the tone at the same time.

Repeat the test on your patient's left mastoid process.

If you suspect your patient has a hearing deficit, recommend she get an audiogram for a more accurate assessment.

Always document the type of test you performed, the result, and the kind of tuning fork used, in your nurses' notes.

Ear inspection

Interpreting Weber, Rinne, or Schwabach tests

Has it been a while since you've had to interpret and document results from Weber, Rinne, or Schwabach tests? If so, study the chart below to refresh your memory. Remember, you'll need the results of all three tests to properly evaluate your patient's hearing.

Test	Normal hearing	Conductive hearing loss	Sensorineural hearing loss
Weber	Patient hears same tone (intensity and volume) in both ears. Document result as Weber negative.	Patient hears the tone louder in the affected ear. Document result as Weber right or Weber left.	The Weber test is inconclusive in this particular condition. However, you may expect the patient to hear the tone equally or louder in the ear you suspect is *unaffected*.
Rinne	Patient hears an air-conducted tone twice as long as a bone-conducted tone. Document result as +R (Rinne positive).	Patient hears a bone-conducted tone for as long or longer than he hears an air-conducted tone. Document result as −R (Rinne negative).	Patient hears air-conducted tones longer than bone-conducted tones. Document result as +R (Rinne positive).
Schwabach	Patient and nurse hear tone for equal amounts of time. Document time in seconds.	Patient hears tone longer than nurse. Document time in seconds.	Nurse hears tone longer than patient. Document time in seconds.

Recognizing common ear problems

DANGER SIGNS

Assessment variables	Acute suppurative otitis media	Acute labyrinthitis	Meniere's syndrome	Acute otitis externa	Otosclerosis
Discharge in external canal	• None (unless eardrum is ruptured)	• None	• None	• Usually yellow and tenacious	• None
Pain	• Severe (a deep throbbing earache is common)	• None	• None	• May be severe (manipulation of auricle and tragus greatly increases pain)	• None
Hearing	• Mild conductive loss	• Sensorineural loss	• Sensorineural loss	• Patient may have either normal hearing or a mild conductive loss.	• Conductive loss increases as condition progresses.
Otoscopic exam	• External ear canal appears normal. • Eardrum looks dull, red, and bulging. • Eardrum may be perforated.	• External ear canal appears normal. • Eardrum looks normal. • If otitis media is also present, expect eardrum to be dull, red, and bulging.	• External ear canal appears normal. • Eardrum appears normal.	• Erythema and edema are present on the external ear canal • Eardrum either looks normal or is red.	• External ear canal appears normal. • Eardrum looks normal.
Vertigo	• None or mild	• Severe (whirling sensation)	• Severe (episodic whirling sensations)	• None or mild	• None
Tinnitus	• Possible	• Present in almost all patients	• Present and constant	• Possible	• Common
Special	• Fever and chills commonly accompany this condition.	• Nausea, vomiting, and nystagmus accompany this condition.	• Nausea and vomiting accompany this condition.	• Adenopathy is present.	• Not applicable

Nose and sinus inspection

Do you know what to look for when you examine a patient's nose or sinuses? Here are some questions to test your knowledge:
• What color is considered normal for the mucous membrane?
• How can you differentiate a nasal polyp from an impacted foreign object in the nose?
• How can you recognize sinuses that are filled with fluid or purulent drainage?

Can you answer these questions completely? If not, or if you have other questions about examining a patient's nose and sinuses, read the following pages.

DOCUMENTING

Nose and sinus questions: What to ask

Preparing to examine your patient's nose and sinuses? Before you begin, interview your patient to gather some baseline information. Here are some questions to ask:
• How would you describe your sense of smell? Can you differentiate one odor from another?
• Do you have any pain or discomfort in your nose and sinuses? If so, can you describe it? When does it occur? Does anything relieve it?
• How frequently do you have a runny nose? When you do, is it at any certain time of day? Is it more frequent during a particular season? Is it usually from one nostril or from both nostrils? What color is the drainage? Does the drainage have an odor?
• Have you ever had sinus trouble? Do you have hay fever or any other allergies? If so, do you take medication to relieve it? What kind?
• Do you ever have nosebleeds? If so, how often? Are they more frequent at a certain season or time of day? Do they follow a pattern? Are you able to stop the bleeding? How?
• Have you ever injured your nose? If so, describe the details.
• Have you ever had surgery on your nose or sinuses? If so, why? When was it?
• Can you describe any other nose or sinus problems you've been having?

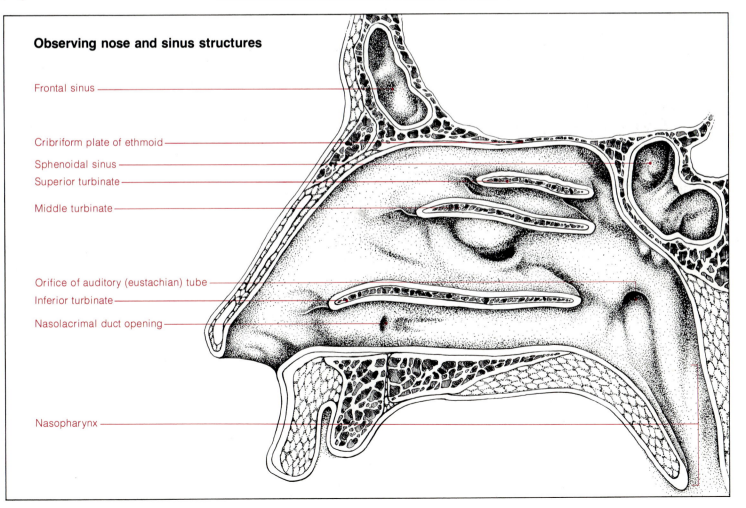

Observing nose and sinus structures

Frontal sinus

Cribriform plate of ethmoid

Sphenoidal sinus

Superior turbinate

Middle turbinate

Orifice of auditory (eustachian) tube

Inferior turbinate

Nasolacrimal duct opening

Nasopharynx

Nose and sinus inspection

Inspecting your patient's nose

1 *Suppose you're inspecting your patient's nose. Do you know what to look for?*

Begin by noting any discharge, inflammation, or deformities. Also, observe the size and shape of your patient's nose. Explain the nasal examination to your patient.

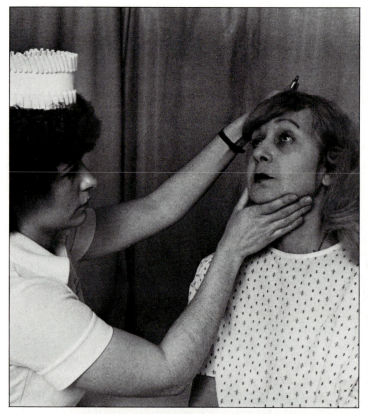

2 Next, shine a penlight into your patient's right nostril, as the nurse is doing here. Make sure the nasal septum's positioned midway between her nostrils. Notice the moist, pink, shiny mucous membrane that covers the interior nasal area.

You may also see the inferior turbinate, which is the lowest of the three mucous membrane-covered bony plates in the nasopharynx (see step 8).

Now, repeat the procedure in the left nostril.

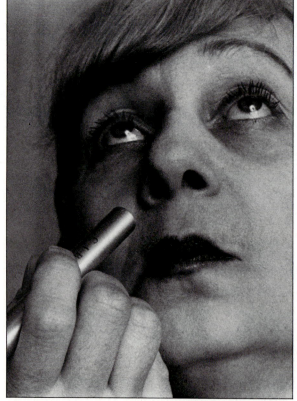

3 Test for nasal obstructions. To do this, ask your patient to hold her left nostril closed. Then, instruct her to exhale through her nose. As she does, note any difficulty.

Repeat this procedure on your patient's right nostril, and compare the results.

🞂 *Nursing tip:* Hold a small mirror under your patient's nostrils (see inset). When she exhales, compare the sizes of the right and left condensation circles that form on the mirror. If you see a difference, your patient may have a nasal obstruction.

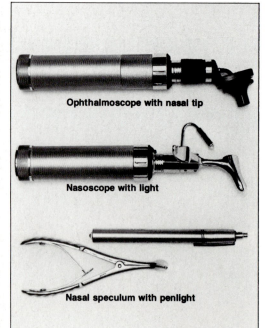

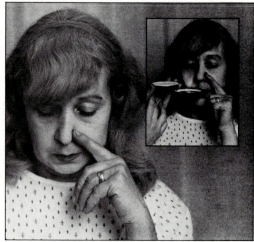

Ophthalmoscope with nasal tip

Nasoscope with light

Nasal speculum with penlight

4 To see the inside of your patient's nose, you'll need a short, broad nasal tip for your ophthalmoscope handle. Or you may use a nasoscope with an attached light, or a nasal speculum with a penlight.

5 Hold the speculum between your thumb and index finger, using your other fingers to control the speculum's spring.

If possible, have your patient rest her head against a wall or other firm support. This will stabilize her head and help prevent injury if she moves.

Insert the scissor-like blades about ½" (1.3 cm) into the nasal vestibule. As you do, place your right index finger on the lower side of your patient's nose to stabilize the blades.

[Inset] Carefully open the blades.

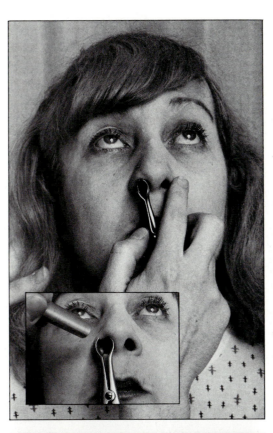

6 If you're using a nasoscope with an attached light, open the blades by pushing down on the lever, as shown here.

[Inset] If you're using an ophthalmoscope with a nasal tip, make sure the tip's securely attached before you insert it in your patient's nose. (For details on assembling and operating the ophthalmoscope, see pages 34 and 35.)

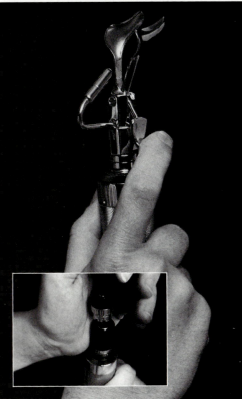

7 When the nasoscope or nasal speculum is properly positioned in your patient's right nostril, examine her nasal septum. If all's well, the septum will look pink and free of any inflammation, swelling, holes, ulcerations, crusting, or sharp edges.

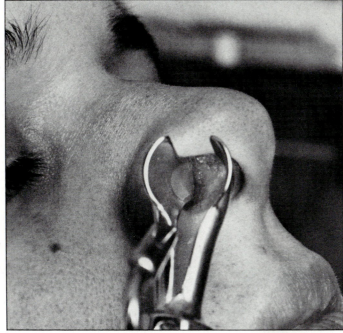

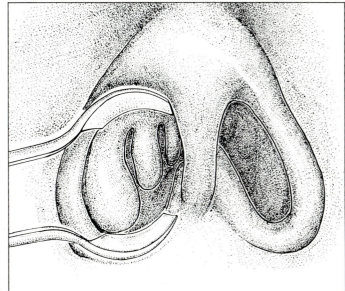

8 Finally, locate the inferior and the middle turbinates. These should appear as curving bony protrusions inside the nose and should be covered by mucous membrane.

If you see any signs of purulent drainage on the turbinates, suspect infection. Also, check for nasal polyps, which are pale, shiny balls attached by stalks to the turbinates.

Repeat this procedure on your patient's left nostril, and document your findings.

Nose and sinus inspection

How to palpate and percuss your patient's sinus areas

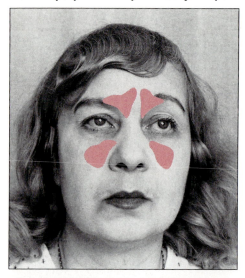

1 *Examining your patient's sinuses? If so, begin by explaining the procedure to your patient. Then, study this photo to locate both her frontal and maxillary sinuses.*

As you know, to properly check the sinuses for fullness and tenderness, you must palpate and percuss the skull areas directly over and below them. Here's how:

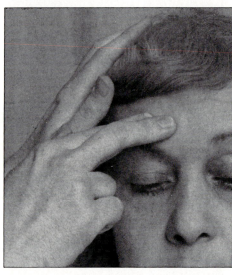

2 Using your fingertips, palpate above the right eyebrow's inner aspect (over frontal sinus), as the nurse is doing here. Note any tenderness or fullness.

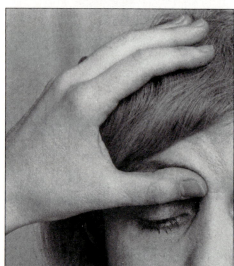

3 Next, using your thumb, palpate the area to the right of your patient's nose, against the bony orbit (below frontal sinus).

Repeat this procedure on your patient's left side. If all's well, your patient will feel equal pressure—but no pain—on top of and below each frontal sinus.

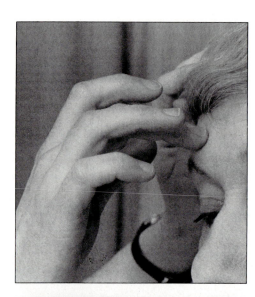

4 Next, percuss the area directly over your patient's frontal sinuses. To do this, gently tap her forehead above her right eyebrow. If everything's OK, you'll hear a hollow sound.

Repeat this procedure on your patient's left frontal sinus.

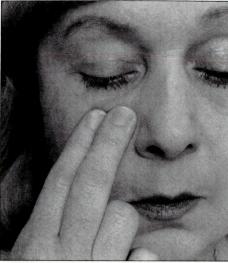

5 Now, gently applying upward pressure, palpate the area directly on top of your patient's right maxillary sinus. Note any fullness or tenderness.

Then, repeat this procedure, palpating your patient's left maxillary sinus.

If all's well, your patient will feel equal pressure—but no pain—on top of each maxillary sinus.

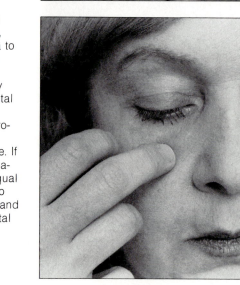

6 Percuss the area over your patient's right maxillary sinus. Note any tenderness or fullness. If everything's OK, you'll hear a hollow sound.

Repeat this procedure on your patient's left maxillary sinus.

Finally, document your findings in your nurses' notes.

How to inspect your patient's sinuses

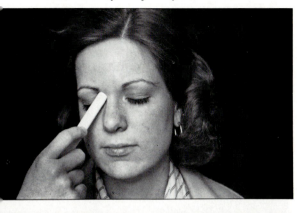

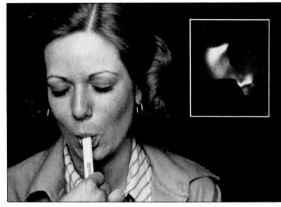

1 *Now, you'll transilluminate your patient's frontal and maxillary sinus structures to check for obstructions and fluid. To do this, you'll need a dark room and a penlight. Then, proceed as follows:*

Examine the frontal sinus structure by gently pressing the penlight against your patient's skin, slightly below the upper rim of the right eye's orbit. Make sure the penlight's facing upward and inward, as shown here.

2 Before you turn on the penlight, shade your patient's eyes by placing your hand below her bony orbit, as shown in this photo.

[Inset] Now, turn on the penlight. If her right frontal sinus contains air, you'll see an illuminated area above her right eyebrow. Then, repeat the test on her left frontal sinus.

Suppose one or both of your patient's frontal sinuses appear dark. The sinuses may be filled with fluid or pus.

3 Now you're ready to transilluminate the maxillary sinuses. If your patient wears upper dentures, ask her to remove them.

Then, position the penlight inside her mouth. Direct the penlight's tip toward her right maxillary sinus. Ask your patient to close her lips.

[Inset] You should see a bright area under your patient's right eye. If you have difficulty seeing this area, shade the lower part of her face. If the sinus still appears dark, it may be filled with fluid or pus.

Now, using the same procedure, transilluminate your patient's left maxillary sinus.

Document your findings. *Important:* A third set of sinuses, the ethmoid sinuses, are located in the roof of your patient's mouth and can't be examined without the use of special instruments or X-rays.

Recognizing common nose problems

DANGER SIGNS

Assessment variables	Epistaxis	Acute nasopharyngitis	Acute suppurative sinusitis	Deviated septum	Allergic rhinitis
Nasal discharge	• Blood	• Purulent	• Purulent (if sinus duct is not obstructed)	• Seldom	• Thin, profuse, and watery
Pain	• None (unless condition was caused by trauma)	• Headache (feeling of fullness behind the nose)	• Severe pain, usually localized. Palpation of involved sinus produces acute pain.	• Patient may either have a headache or be pain free.	• Frontal headache is common.
Nasoscopic exam	• Shows exact site of bloody discharge, which will probably be in the anterior part of the nasal septum	• Inflamed posterior mucous membrane evident, with characteristic yellow or white follicles	• Edematous mucosa present in involved meatus.	• Septum inclines toward one side or toward both sides, forming an S shape	• Mucosa appears smooth and shiny. • Turbinates look pale and engorged.
Special	• None	• Patient may have fever and postnasal drip.	• Patient has fever and postnasal drip.	• Patient may have trouble breathing through his nose.	• Patient usually sneezes and has tearing, itchy eyes. • Nasal polyps are common when condition is chronic.

Mouth and throat inspection

Are you inspecting your patient's mouth and throat? If so, do you know how to check her teeth for nerve damage? How to use a laryngeal mirror properly?

The next few pages will take you step by step through a mouth and throat exam. Study the photostory and illustrations carefully. They'll help you learn how to differentiate a normal mouth and throat condition from an abnormal one.

DOCUMENTING

**Mouth and throat questions:
What to ask**

Whenever you examine your patient's mouth and throat, you'll want baseline data to refer to. Study the sample questions below. They'll give you an idea of what you'll want to include in your interview.

• Rate your sense of taste. Is it excellent? Good? Fair? Or poor? Are you able to distinguish one flavor from another? Have you noticed any change in your ability to taste? Or any peculiarities?
• Do you have any problems chewing or swallowing food?
• Describe the condition of your teeth. When was your last dental exam? What did the dentist find? Did you have any cavities or infections? When was your last set of oral X-rays taken?
• Do you have any loose or missing teeth? If so, which ones? How long have they been loose or missing?
• Do you wear dentures? If so, how long have you been wearing them? How do they fit? Do you use dental adhesive?
• How do your gums feel? Do they bleed? Do you have sores on your gums or tongue?
• Have you noticed any bleeding from your mouth? If so, when?
• Do you have any problems speaking? If so, describe the details. Do you get tongue-tied?
• Do you have hoarseness or scratchiness in your voice? If so, when did you first notice this?
• How does your throat usually feel? When was your last sore throat? How many sore throats do you have yearly? Do you take anything to relieve them?
• Have you ever been treated for tonsillitis or strep throat? If so, describe the details.
• Have you ever had a broken jaw or an injury to your mouth or teeth? If so, describe the details.
• Have you had any type of oral surgery? If so, describe the details.
• Do you smoke? How many cigars or packs of cigarettes do you smoke a day? Do you smoke a pipe?
• Have you noticed any other problems?

Viewing mouth and throat structures

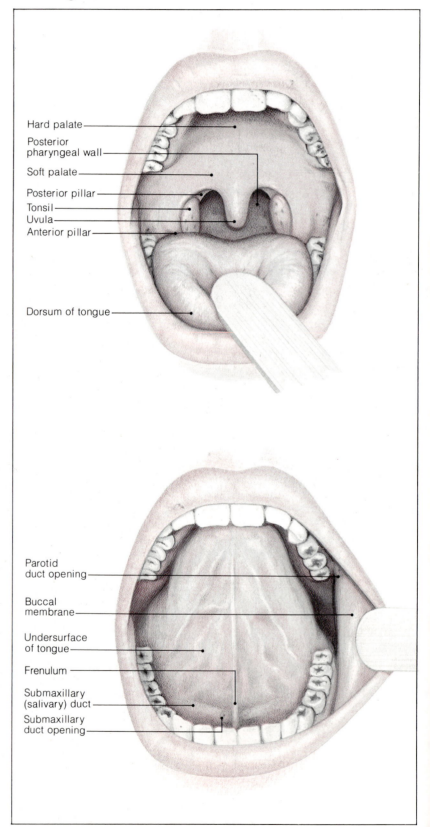

Hard palate

Posterior pharyngeal wall

Soft palate

Posterior pillar

Tonsil

Uvula

Anterior pillar

Dorsum of tongue

Parotid duct opening

Buccal membrane

Undersurface of tongue

Frenulum

Submaxillary (salivary) duct

Submaxillary duct opening

Inspecting your patient's mouth

1 *Preparing to examine your patient's mouth? You'll need a gauze pad, tongue depressor, penlight, glove or finger cot, and a laryngeal mirror with an attached light.*

Thoroughly explain the examination to your patient. Does she seem cooperative? If she doesn't, don't put your fingers in her mouth. Instead, use a tongue depressor.

If your patient has dentures, ask her to remove them. Also, remove any lipstick she may be wearing. Then, follow these steps:

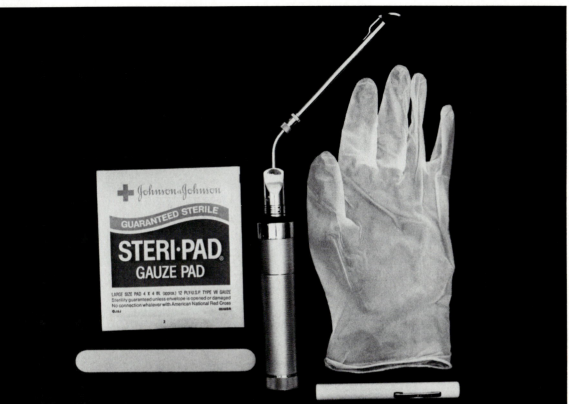

2 First, inspect your patient's lips. They should be pink and smooth. Wearing a glove or finger cot, palpate her lips for ulcers, nodules, or lesions. If you find any, note their size and hardness.

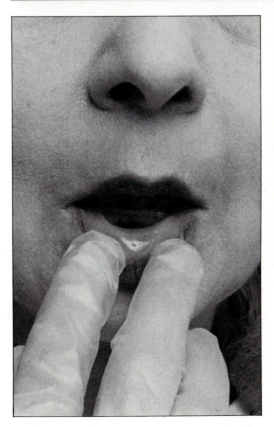

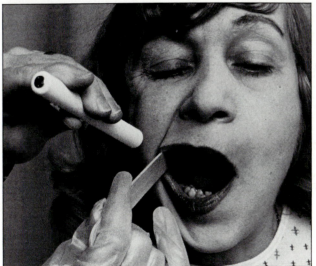

3 Now, ask your patient to open her mouth. Use a tongue depressor to gently push out her right cheek. Then, check her gums. They should be pink and moist. Note any inflammation, swelling, bleeding, retraction, or distortion.

Locate her parotid duct, which is located inside the cheek, opposite the second molars. Note any inflammation or drainage.

Repeat the entire procedure on your patient's left side, and document your findings.

Mouth and throat inspection

Inspecting your patient's mouth continued

4 Next, look at your patient's teeth. Unless she's had dental problems, she should have 32 teeth—8 on each side of her upper and lower jaws.

Using the tongue depressor, tap each tooth, both upper and lower, on her right side. If everything's OK, your patient will feel a tapping sensation in each tooth.

If your patient complains of pain, she may have an abscess. Suppose your patient doesn't feel *any* sensation. Suspect nerve damage.

Repeat the procedure on her left side.

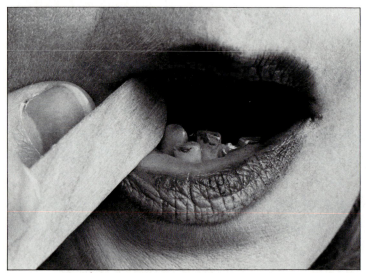

6 Now, ask your patient to lightly close her mouth and relax her lips. Check her bite by retracting her upper and lower lips, as shown here.

Your patient's molars and premolars should meet. Also, her lower canines and incisors should slide slightly inside her upper front teeth.

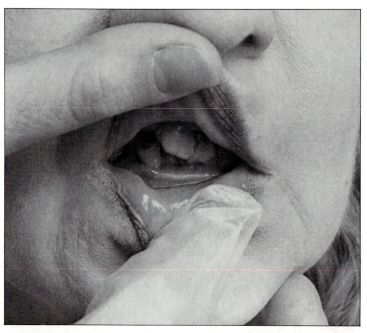

5 Next, note any missing teeth. Also look for broken or severely decayed teeth. If a tooth looks loose, check it by wobbling it with your finger or a tongue depressor.

Important: If you find an extremely loose tooth, suggest to your patient that it be extracted. If she takes your suggestion, ask a trained health-care professional to extract the tooth, as soon as possible.

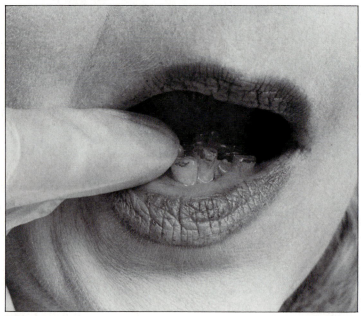

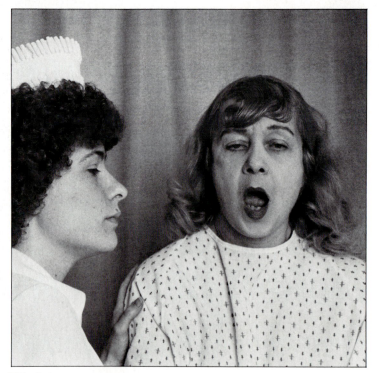

7 Ask your patient to yawn. As she yawns, listen for noises in her jaw joints. If you hear anything—for example, a clicking sound—your patient may have arthritis or degeneration of the jaw.

8 While your patient's mouth is wide open, use a tongue depressor to push her right cheek out.

With a penlight, check the upper, lower, and middle buccal membranes inside her right cheek. If everything's OK, you'll see smooth, pink pigmentation. However, if your patient's black, you'll see patchy pink pigmentation.

Palpate any ulcers, growths, or lesions you may find, and note their size and hardness. Document your findings.

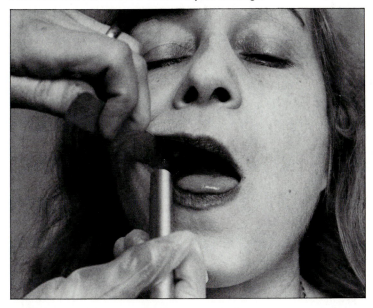

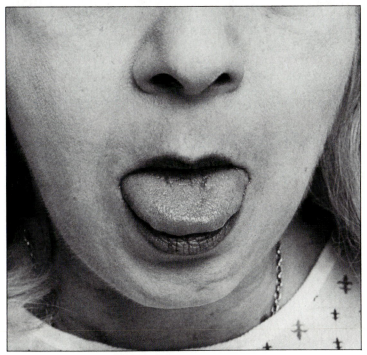

9 Next, ask your patient to stick out her tongue. It should look velvety and pink. Pay particular attention to the tip and sides of her tongue. Palpate any ulcers, growths, or lesions you may find, noting size and hardness.

10 Ask your patient to put the tip of her tongue on the roof of her mouth. Then, check under her tongue. The mucous membrane should be pink, moist, and smooth. Palpate any ulcers, growths, or lesions you may find, noting size and hardness.

[Inset] At the same time you're checking the mucous membrane, palpate your patient's submaxillary (salivary) ducts, which are located on either side of the frenulum. The area should feel soft and moist. Note any hardness or irregularities, and document them.

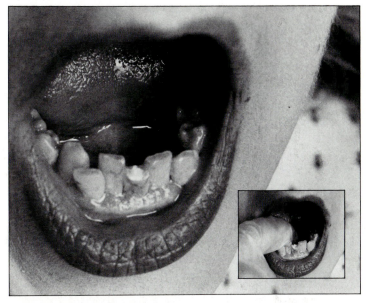

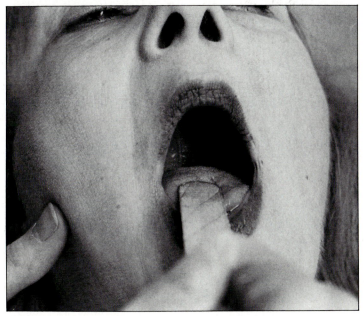

11 Finally, shine a penlight at the roof of your patient's mouth. To do this, you may have to hold her tongue down with a tongue depressor. If everything's OK, the hard palate will be firm and white. The soft palate will appear pink and cushiony.

Document your findings in your nurses' notes.

Now you're ready to examine your patient's throat, as explained on page 62.

Mouth and throat inspection

Examining your patient's throat

1 *Are you assessing your patient's throat? If so, hold your patient's tongue down with a tongue depressor and ask him to pronounce a vowel; for example, Ah.* As he does, locate the uvula, which should be smooth and pink. If it appears red or swollen, your patient may be having an allergic reaction. Suppose you see a bifid uvula. Your patient may have a submucous cleft palate.

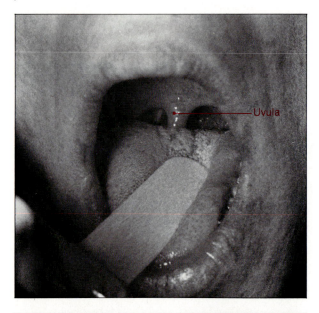

2 Now, locate the fauces, which is the folded tense tissue at the back of his mouth.

Look for the tonsils on either side of the fauces. If everything's OK, the tonsils will look like mottled brown or pink cushions of tissue.

Behind the fauces, you'll see the pharynx, which should look pink and smooth in nonsmokers and yellowish-red (with small nodules) in smokers.

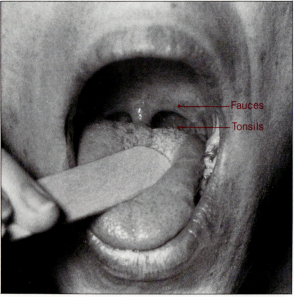

3 Next, tilt your patient's head backward. Insert the laryngeal mirror along the side of his mouth, with the mirror pointing up.

Important: If you have difficulty inserting the mirror because of your patient's gag reflex, get a doctor's order for anesthetic throat spray. Then, reinsert the mirror.

Shine the light into your patient's throat to check his posterior nasal cavity (see the illustration). Because the mirror is small, you'll only be able to see one portion of the cavity at a time.

If all's well, the nasal cavity will be unobstructed.

Nursing tip: To prevent the mirror from fogging, spray it with an antifog solution.

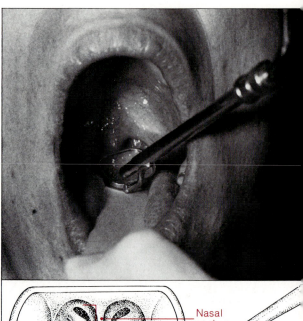

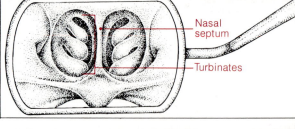

4 Next, examine your patient's larynx and vocal cords. To do this, angle the laryngeal mirror down your patient's throat. Rest the bent part of the mirror just above his uvula. Locate the pink, moist epiglottis, as shown in the illustration. Note any swelling, ulcerations, or growths, and document them.

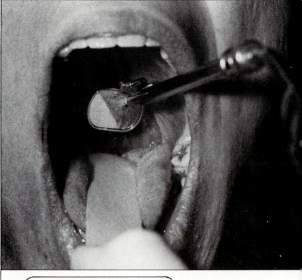

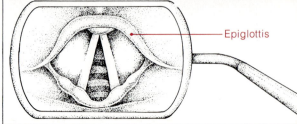

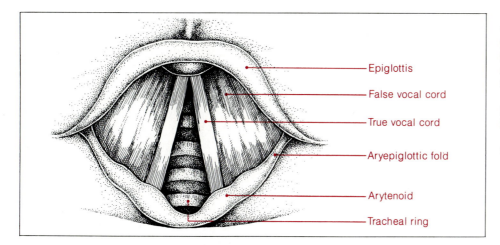

- Epiglottis
- False vocal cord
- True vocal cord
- Aryepiglottic fold
- Arytenoid
- Tracheal ring

5 Now ask your patient to say *Ah* or *Eee*. As he does, you'll see both the false and the true vocal cords, as shown in this illustration. Expect your patient's vocal cords to open outward as he inhales and inward as he exhales.

Check their appearance. They should look smooth, white, and glistening. Note any ulcers, inflammation, discharge, or growths.

When you've completed the examination, document all your findings.

DANGER SIGNS

Detecting mouth and throat problems

Assessment variables	Oral herpes labiales (herpes simplex)	Oral leukoplakia	Acute pharyngitis	Acute tonsillitis	Cancer of larynx
Discharge	• Clear yellow (if vesicle breaks)	• None	• Pus or yellow exudate on throat's mucous membrane	• Pus or yellow exudate on tonsils	• None
Pain	• Burning and itchiness common before vesicle forms. • After vesicle forms, discomfort at lesion site common.	• Only in advanced stages of the condition	• Varies from slight scratchiness to severe throat pain (in strep throat)	• Sore throat, varying in severity	• Only in advanced stages of the condition
Difficulty swallowing	• None	• None	• Mild to severe	• Some difficulty possible	• Late symptom of condition
Oral examination	• Clear vesicles formed on slightly elevated reddened tissue (this usually occurs at junction of lip mucosa and skin) • Following rupture, lesion appears yellow and encrusted.	• Patches of various sizes and shapes may be found in mouth. • Patches may be yellow white or gray white. • When palpated, patches usually feel thickened and leathery. • Patches may be ulcerated or fissured.	• Pharyngeal mucous membrane appears swollen and reddened. • If strep throat present, membrane may be dotted with yellow follicles.	• Tonsils enlarged and red • If strep throat is present, tonsils may be dotted with yellow follicles.	• Laryngeal mirror exam reveals a lesion on the true vocal cord or elsewhere on the larynx. (Character of the lesion will vary. Diagnosis of cancer must be based on biopsy results.)
Special	None	None	• Hacking cough • If strep throat is present, patient may also have high fever, chills, headache, and muscular aches.	• Anterior cervical lymph glands may be swollen and tender. • Fever, chills, and muscular aches	• Hoarseness (first symptom of vocal cord malignancy) • Pain on swallowing may be later sign of a malignancy elsewhere on the larynx.

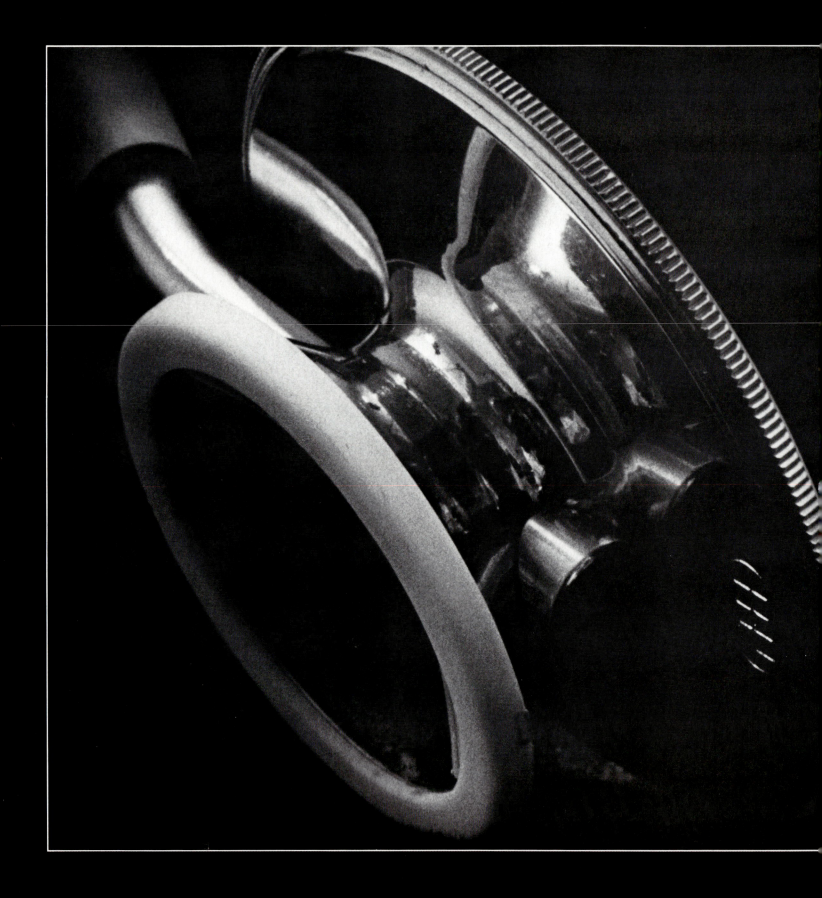

Examining the Thorax

Observation and inspection

Respiratory system

Cardiovascular system

Observation and inspection

When's the last time you taught a patient how to examine her breasts? Or assessed her respiratory rate? Or inspected her thorax?

If it's been a while, study the next few pages to refresh your memory. In them, you'll find the step-by-step guidelines you need...plus much, much more.

How to inspect your patient's thorax

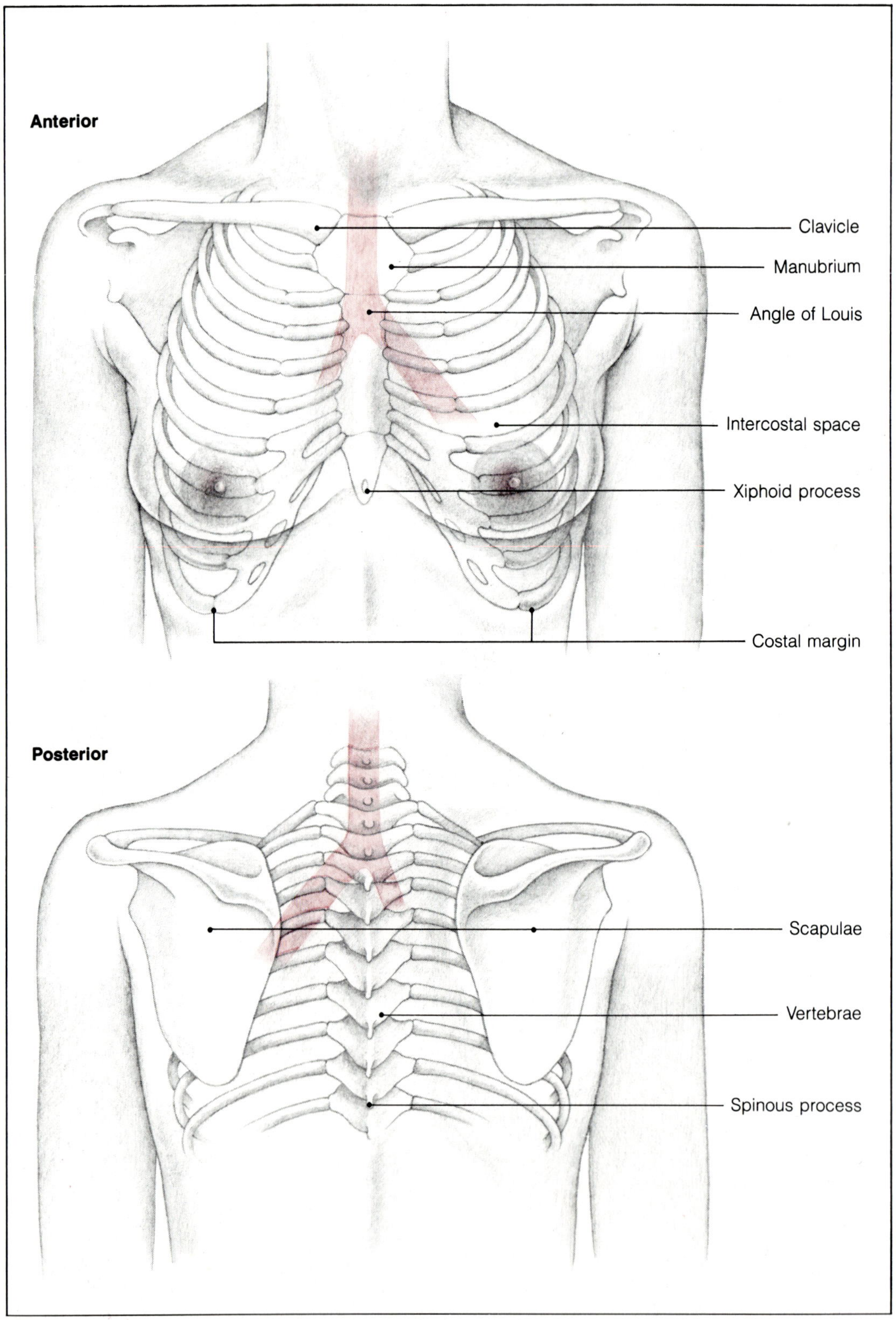

Anterior

- Clavicle
- Manubrium
- Angle of Louis
- Intercostal space
- Xiphoid process
- Costal margin

Posterior

- Scapulae
- Vertebrae
- Spinous process

1 *Are you inspecting your patient's thorax? If so, follow these steps:* First, familiarize yourself with the thoracic landmarks shown in these illustrations. Then, locate these landmarks on your patient's anterior and posterior chest.

2 Observe your patient from her right side. Her anteroposterior chest should appear symmetrical and elliptical.

Observe her lateral chest. Expect her anterior ribs to slope downward.

Now, look at the inset illustration, and do your best to compare your patient's chest to it. (Or, use a chest depth caliper.) As you can see, the diameter of her chest should be less than her lateral chest diameter.

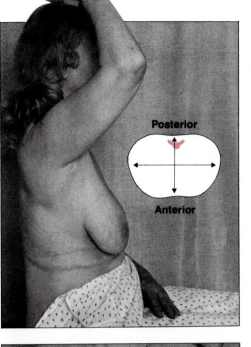

3 Inspect the skin on your patient's anterior and posterior chest. (If your patient's a female, check under her breasts.) Look for any skin discolorations, scars, dimpling, lesions, lumps, or ulcerations, noting location and color.

Observe any chest hair your patient may have, and record the type, pattern, and amount.

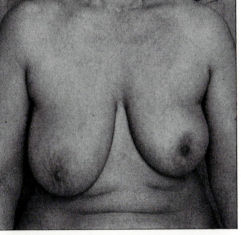

4 Now, palpate your patient's anterior and posterior chest, noting skin temperature and moistness. Be sure to palpate any scars, dimpling, lesions, lumps, or ulcerations you may have observed, and note their texture. Also, palpate any pulsations occurring away from the heart area, and record their location, force, and frequency.

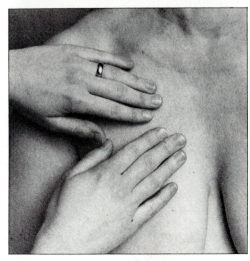

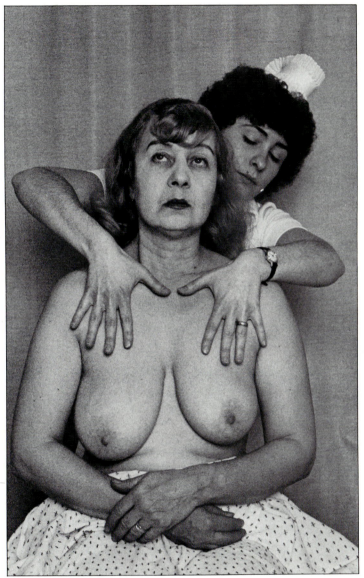

5 Next, stand behind your patient, as the nurse is doing here. Reach over her shoulders, and place your palms on her upper chest. Position your thumbs directly over her sternum, and spread your fingers so they extend downward and to the sides. Ask your patient to take a deep breath and exhale. If all's well, you'll feel her thoracic wall expand evenly and equally. Her shoulders should rise *slightly* during inspiration and fall *slightly* during expiration.

Note any asymmetrical expansion or use of accessory muscles during respiration. Either may indicate lung congestion, flail chest, pneumothorax, or pain on the affected side.

Then, observe your patient's breathing patterns. Be sure to count her respiratory rate for a full minute. If everything's OK, your patient's respiratory rate will be between 12 and 20 breaths per minute. (For more information on assessing your patient's respiratory system, see pages 71 to 81.)

Note any signs of respiratory distress; for example, labored breathing, cyanosis, anxiety, or tachycardia.

Finally, document all your findings in your nurses' notes.

Observation and inspection

Identifying common chest deviations

As you observe and inspect your patient's thorax, you may notice deviations in its size or shape. As you know, these deviations may help. you detect other problems your patient may have.

Use this chart as a guide in identifying chest deviations.

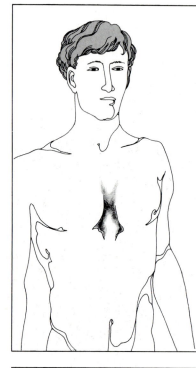

PECTUS EXCAVATUM
(funnel chest)

Physical appearance
• Sinking or funnel-shaped depression of lower sternum; diminished anteroposterior chest diameter

Possible cause
• Unknown but may be from unbalanced growth in costo-chrondral regions during fetal development

Signs and associated conditions
• Postural disorders; for example, forward displacement of neck and shoulders
• Upper thoracic kyphosis
• Protuberant abdomen
• Functional heart murmur

Treatment
• If surgery is performed during first 7 years of life, condition may be corrected.

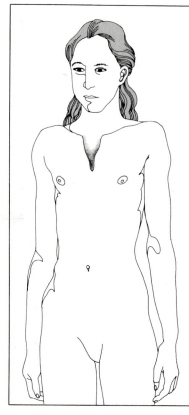

BIFID STERNUM

Physical appearance
• Complete or incomplete sternal separation

Possible cause
• Sternal bands fail to fuse during fetal development.

Signs and associated conditions
• Missing or supernumerary ribs
• Ectopia cordis (development of heart outside thoracic cavity)

Treatment
• If sternal separation is complete, sternum my be joined surgically, possibly with a prosthesis or a cartilage autograft.
• If sternal separation is *incomplete,* condition may be corrected surgically.

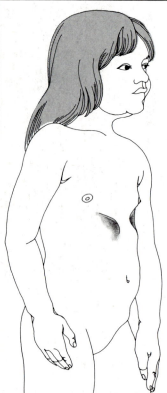

PECTUS CARINATUM
(pigeon breast, chicken breast, or keeled breast)

Physical appearance
• Projection of sternum beyond abdomen's frontal plane. Evident in two variations: chondro-manubrial (projection greatest at xiphoid process) and chondro-gladiolar (projection greatest at or near center of sternum).

Possible cause
• Unknown but may be from excessive cartilage growth during fetal development

Signs and associated conditions
• Functional cardiac or pulmonary disorders

Treatment
• For cosmetic reasons, condition may be corrected surgically.

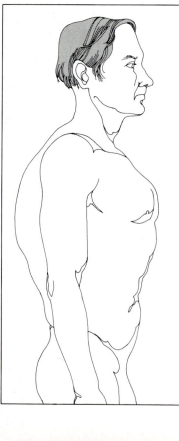

BARREL CHEST

Physical appearance
• Enlarged anteroposterior and transverse chest dimensions (chest appears barrel-shaped)
• Ribs usually appear more horizontal than sloped.

Possible cause
• Emphysema. Because lungs are constantly overexpanded, chest becomes rigid and ribs become fixed at joints.

Signs and associated conditions
• Increasing shortness of breath
• Chronic cough
• Wheezing

Treatment
• If barrel chest is fully developed, condition can't be corrected surgically.
• If condition is detected in early stage, treatment is directed at underlying pathology.

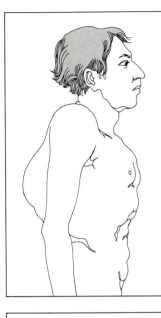

KYPHOSIS

Physical appearance
• Rounded shoulders and exaggerated posterior chest convexity (hunchback)

Possible causes
• Poor posture
• Tuberculosis
• Chronic arthritis
• Compression fractures of thoracic vertebrae

Signs and associated conditions
• Poor posture
• As condition develops, pulmonary function decreases.

Treatment
• If detected early, condition may be corrected with exercise and patient education on good posture.
• In advanced stage, condition may be corrected with braces or surgery.

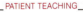

SCOLIOSIS

Physical appearance
• Spine curves from left to right (S-shaped spine)

Possible cause
• Condition may be idiopathic or from a deformity of one or more vertebrae.

Signs and associated conditions
• Poor posture
• Decreased pulmonary function
• As condition progresses, patient has decreased reflexes and altered motor function in legs.

Treatment
• Condition may be treated with exercise, a brace, or a splint.
• Condition may be corrected surgically by anterior or posterior spinal fusion.

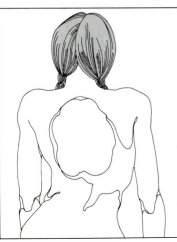

KYPHOSCOLIOSIS

Physical appearance
• Rounded shoulders, exaggerated thoracic convexity, and left-to-right spinal curvature (combination of kyphosis and scoliosis)

Possible cause
• See kyphosis and scoliosis.

Signs and associated conditions
• If condition is severe, patient may have cardiopulmonary failure.
• If condition is mild, patient may be asymptomatic.

Treatment
• See kyphosis and scoliosis.

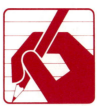

Breast questions: What to ask

Whether your patient is male or female, you'll want to gather some baseline information before you do a breast examination. Here are some questions you may want to ask:
• Have you noticed any lumps or soreness in your breasts? If so, when?
• (For female patients) Do you notice lumps or soreness before, during, or after your menstrual period?
• Do you ever have any secretions or discharge from your nipples? If so, when? Describe the color and consistency.
• Do you have any soreness or ulcerations around your nipples? If so, describe the details.
• Have you ever had mammography?
• Has anyone in your family had breast cancer?
• Have you had any type of breast surgery? If so, when? Describe the details.
• Do you have any other problems with your breasts?

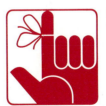

Performing a breast exam

Whenever you examine your patient's breasts, stress the importance of performing a self-examination on a regular basis.

Explain the purposes of the exam: looking for changes in the shape and size of the breasts, checking for nipple secretions, and feeling for any masses or thickening in the breast area. Remind your patient that lumps or irregularities in the breast area aren't necessarily cancerous but should be checked by a doctor.

Now, using the steps on the next page as a guideline, examine your patient's breasts. Explain each step to her as you do it. Then give her a copy of the following home care aid.

Important: Remember to examine your male patient's breasts also, especially if he's receiving hormone therapy.

Patient teaching

Home care
How to examine your breasts

Dear Patient:

1 As you know, examining your breasts regularly is one way you can detect breast cancer early. By doing the examination at least once a month, (after your menstrual period is best), you'll become more familiar with your breasts. You should be able to recognize anything abnormal.

Here's how to perform a breast exam: First, sit or stand in front of a mirror, with your arms at your sides. Look for the following: changes in the size or shape of your breasts, skin puckering or dimpling, or nipple secretions. Then, put your arms over your head, and repeat your check.

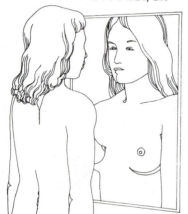

2 Now, lie down, with a pillow or rolled up towel under your right shoulder. Place your right hand behind your head. Put your left hand on the top part of your right breast toward the center of your chest (breastbone).

Moving your fingertips in a small, circular, clockwise motion, feel the top part of your breast from the breastbone to the nipple area.

3 Using the same circular motion, feel the lower part of your breast from the center of your chest to the nipple area. Don't panic if you feel a ridge of firm flesh or tissue in this area. It's perfectly normal.

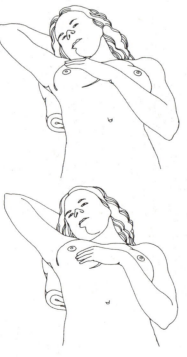

4 Next, use the flat part of your fingertips to feel under your right armpit.

5 Now, with the same circular, clockwise motion as before, feel the upper part of your breast from the nipple area to your right side.

6 Then, feel the lower part of your breast from your right side to your nipple area.

Next, feel your nipple and the surrounding area.

7 Now, bring your right arm to your side and repeat steps 2 through 6.

Finally, repeat the entire examination on your left breast. If you notice abnormalities or changes in either breast, notify your doctor immediately.

Respiratory system

To assess your patient's pulmonary system completely, you'll need to palpate, percuss, and auscultate her lung fields. On the following pages, we'll show you how to competently assess your patient's lungs using these techniques. You'll also find tips on:
• choosing a stethoscope
• evaluating fremitus
• identifying percussion sounds.

Are you familiar with these specifics? If you're not sure, the next few pages will give you the details.

Pulmonary landmarks (anterior and posterior views)

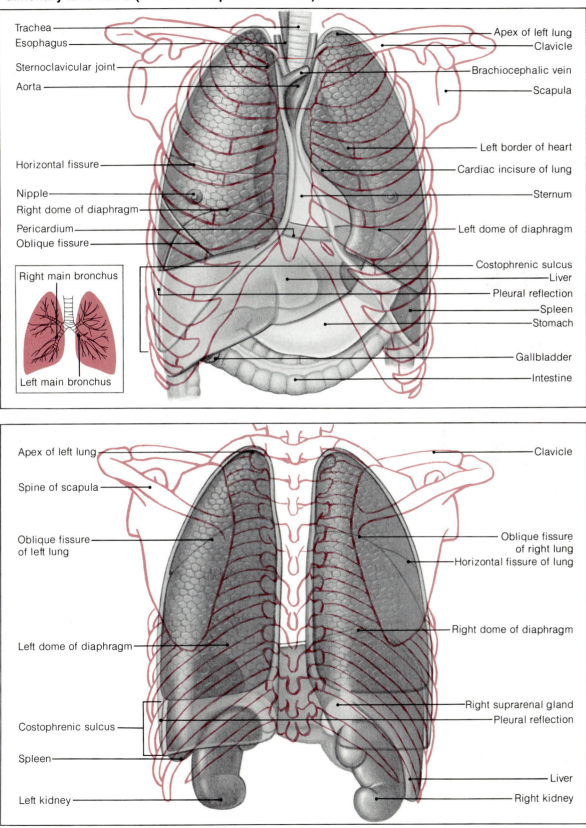

Trachea
Esophagus
Sternoclavicular joint
Aorta
Horizontal fissure
Nipple
Right dome of diaphragm
Pericardium
Oblique fissure

Right main bronchus
Left main bronchus

Apex of left lung
Clavicle
Brachiocephalic vein
Scapula
Left border of heart
Cardiac incisure of lung
Sternum
Left dome of diaphragm
Costophrenic sulcus
Liver
Pleural reflection
Spleen
Stomach
Gallbladder
Intestine

Apex of left lung
Spine of scapula
Oblique fissure of left lung
Left dome of diaphragm
Costophrenic sulcus
Spleen
Left kidney

Clavicle
Oblique fissure of right lung
Horizontal fissure of lung
Right dome of diaphragm
Right suprarenal gland
Pleural reflection
Liver
Right kidney

Respiratory system

**Respiratory
questions:
What to ask**

Before you can inspect and assess
your patient's lungs effectively, you
must find out all you can about her
past and present lung conditions.
You must also collect any specific
information that may indicate future problems. Do you know what
questions to ask? If not, use the
samples below as a guide.
• Have you ever had trouble
breathing? Do you ever have a
shortness of breath? When does
it occur? How long does it take
for your breathing to return to normal?
• Do you have a cough? If so,
when did it start? Do you take anything for it? Do you cough anything up? How much do you
usually cough up? What color is
it? Have you ever coughed up
blood? If so, how often? How was
the condition treated?
• Have you ever been treated for
a lung problem? If so, when? What
type of lung problem was it? When
did it start? Describe the details.
• Do you have any allergies? What
kind? Do you ever wheeze? If so,
when? Do you take any medications for your allergies? What are
they?
• Have you ever had a blood clot
in your lungs? When? Describe
the details.
• Have you ever been exposed
to tuberculosis? If so, when was
your last tuberculin test? Have you
ever had tuberculosis? If so, when?
Were you treated for it?
• When was your last chest X-ray
taken? Was it normal?
• Do you smoke cigarettes, a
pipe, or cigars? If you smoke cigarettes, how many packs a day?
How long have you been smoking? If you no longer smoke, how
long ago did you quit?
• Do you work around chemicals
or fumes? If so, describe what kind.
Explain what contact you have with
these materials.
• Do you work around asbestos,
dust, or coal? If so, describe your
work environment.
• Do you have any other lung
problems?

Palpating lung fields

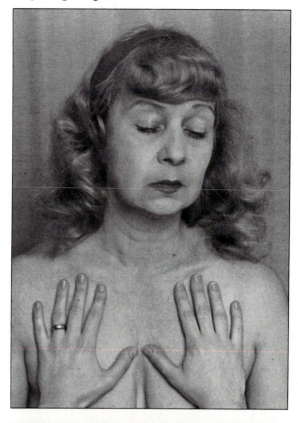

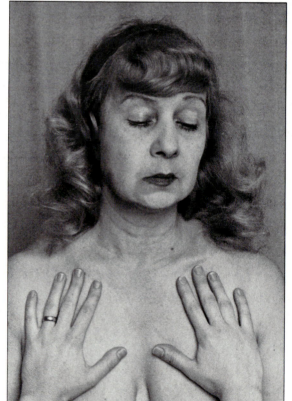

1 Palpation will help you detect lesions, obstructions,
and other abnormalities in your
patient's lungs. Do you know
how to palpate, and to evaluate
your findings properly? If you're
unsure, study the guidelines
in this photostory.

First, seat your patient on the
exam table, with her feet dangling over the side. Then, place
your hands on her upper chest,
as shown in this photo. Make
sure your fingertips rest on her
clavicle and your thumbs meet
over her sternum.

2 Now, ask your patient to
take a deep breath. As she
inhales, hold your fingertips
in place, but let your palms follow the movement of her chest.
If all's well, your thumbs will
move an equal distance apart.

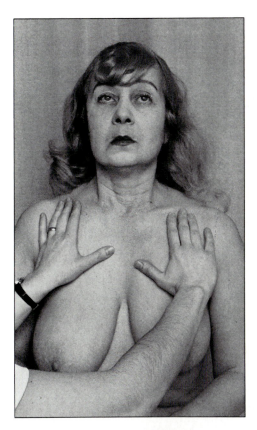

3 If your hands move apart asymmetrically, as in this photo, suspect a lesion or pleural thickening in one of the lungs' upper lobes. Or your patient may have atelectasis, an obstructed bronchus, a misplaced endotracheal tube, a pneumothorax, or pain on the affected side.

As you palpate other areas, note any asymmetrical movement, tenderness, lumps, or masses. A crackling feeling under your patient's skin may indicate subcutaneous emphysema.

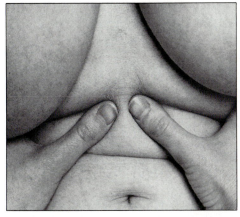

4 Next, check your patient's lung excursion at mid and lower chest. To do this, place your hands on the sides of her chest. Now, draw your thumbs together until they meet below her sternum. As you do, apply gentle pressure to draw a small fold of skin toward the sternum.

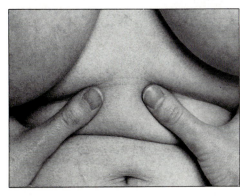

5 Then, ask your patient to take a deep breath. Do your hands move apart symmetrically? If they don't, document the variation in your nurses' notes.

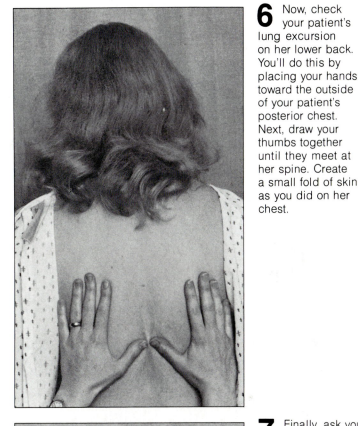

6 Now, check your patient's lung excursion on her lower back. You'll do this by placing your hands toward the outside of your patient's posterior chest. Next, draw your thumbs together until they meet at her spine. Create a small fold of skin, as you did on her chest.

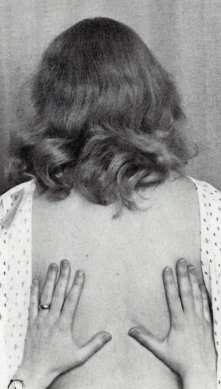

7 Finally, ask your patient to take a deep breath. As she does, your thumbs should move equally apart. If you notice any variation, document it in your nurses' notes.

Respiratory system

How to palpate for tactile fremitus

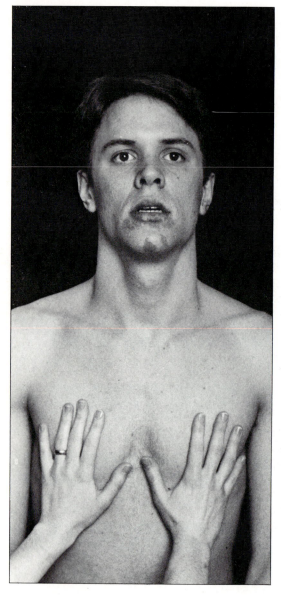

Do you know how to palpate for tactile fremitus properly? If you're unsure, follow the guidelines below. As you know, tactile fremitus is the vibration you feel in your patient's body when he speaks.

First, place your palms lightly on either side of your patient's anterior chest, as shown at left. Then, ask him to repeat a resonant phrase—for example, "ninety-nine"—loudly enough to produce palpable vibrations in his chest.

As you know, if your patient can't speak loudly enough to produce these vibrations, no information can be gained from this test. Also, if your patient's a female, you may be unable to evaluate tactile fremitus on her anterior chest, since breast tissue usually dampens palpable vibrations.

If everything's OK, you'll feel equal vibrations on both sides of your patient's chest.

Suppose you continue to feel fremitus after your patient stops speaking. Suspect abnormalities in your patient's lungs. (For more information on lung abnormalities, see the chart on page 81.)

Continue to palpate your patient's anterior chest following percussion steps on pages 75 and 76. Then, palpate your patient's posterior chest, as shown in photo at the right.

Document your findings in your nurses' notes.

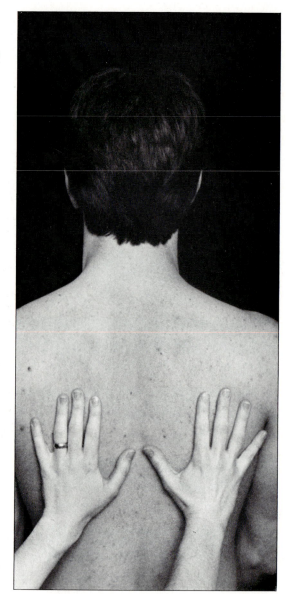

MINI-ASSESSMENT

Evaluating fremitus

We've shown you how to palpate for tactile fremitus. Now, we'll explain how to evaluate your findings. Study this chart carefully.

Findings	Indications
More intense on one side	• Tissue consolidation on the affected side
Less intense on one side	• Emphysema, pneumothorax, or pleural effusion
Absent or faint in upper chest	• Bronchial obstruction or fluid-filled pleural space

Percussing lung fields

1 *Percussing your patient's lungs? Seat your patient on the side of the bed or on an exam table, and make sure the room's at a comfortable temperature.*

Note: In some situations, you may find it easier to percuss your patient's lungs if she lies flat on a bed or an exam table. Explain the examining procedure to her, and ensure her privacy. Then, follow these steps:

First, percuss your patient's anterior chest, above the right clavicle, keeping your finger strikes uniform.

Then, continue percussing until you can identify the sound you hear. If you're having difficulty doing this, study the chart on page 76.

2 Now, continue to percuss your patient's anterior chest, following the sequence shown in this photo. Make sure you percuss between her ribs, *not on them,* or you'll hear bone sounds rather than lung sounds. If everything's OK, you'll hear resonance over most of the lung fields. However, when you percuss over organs, you'll hear a change in sound; for example, dullness over the cardiac area and tympany over the stomach. (The illustration on page 71 shows you where you can expect these sound changes.)

3 Suppose you're percussing a female patient with large breasts. To get an accurate sound, ask her to hold her breasts up or toward the side as you percuss the breast area.

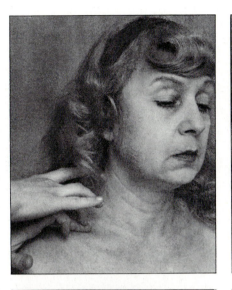

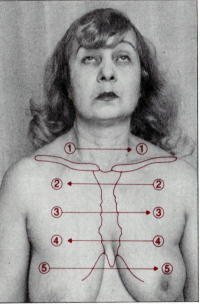

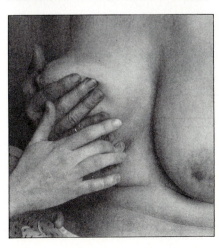

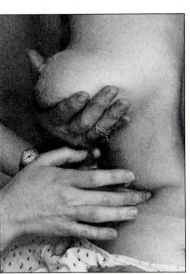

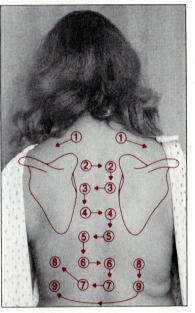

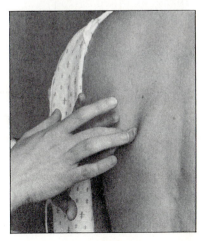

4 Now, percuss downward until the sound changes. For example, on your patient's right side, expect the sound to change from resonant to dull as you percuss over her liver. On her left side, expect it to change from resonant to tympanic as you percuss over her stomach.

5 Now, percuss your patient's posterior chest, following the sequence shown here. Listen for sound variations as you compare one side to the other. If you hear dull sounds, suspect fluid or consolidation in the lung. Document any abnormal sounds you hear in your nurses' notes. Describe them carefully, and include their location.

6 Percuss toward the patient's lower posterior chest (below the scapulae). Expect the sound to change from resonant to dull when you reach the area over the diaphragm.

Respiratory system

Percussing lung fields continued

7 When you locate the diaphragm, measure the diaphragmatic excursion. To do this, ask your patient to take a deep breath. Then, ask her to exhale completely. Tell her to hold her breath as long as possible. Percuss the area until you hear a dull sound, indicating the position of the diaphragm at full *expiration*. Use a marking pen or stick-on dots to mark this location on both sides of her chest.

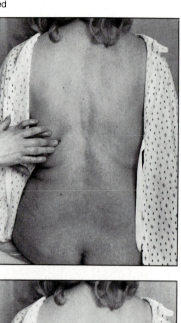

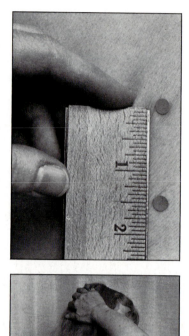

9 Now, measure the distance between the marks on each side, and compare the measurement. The distance should be about 1¼" to 2" (3 to 5 cm) long, and both sides should be almost equal in length.

8 Now, ask your patient to inhale deeply and to hold her breath as long as possible. Percuss until you locate the diaphragm at the point of full *inspiration*. In the same manner as above, mark this location on both sides of her chest.

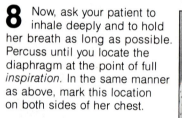

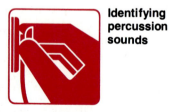

10 Finally, ask your patient to rest her arm on her head, as shown here. Then, percuss her side, along her midaxillary line, at 2" (5 cm) intervals. Repeat the procedure on the opposite side.
  Document your findings in your nurses' notes.

MINI-ASSESSMENT

Identifying percussion sounds

How familiar are you with the various percussion sounds? Do you know what these sounds indicate? If you're unsure, read this chart.

Sound	Pitch	Intensity	Quality	Indication
Resonance	Low	Moderate to loud	Hollow	Normal lung
Hyperresonance	Low	Loud	Booming	Emphysematous lung or pneumothorax
Tympany	High	Loud	Musical, drumlike	Stomach area, abdomen distended with air
Dullness	High	Soft	Thudlike	Liver area, cardiac area, diaphragm, or pleural effusion
Flatness	High	Soft	Extreme dullness	Sternum or atelectic lung

Choosing the right stethoscope

Before you select a stethoscope, carefully consider which model suits your needs. This photo shows some options available.

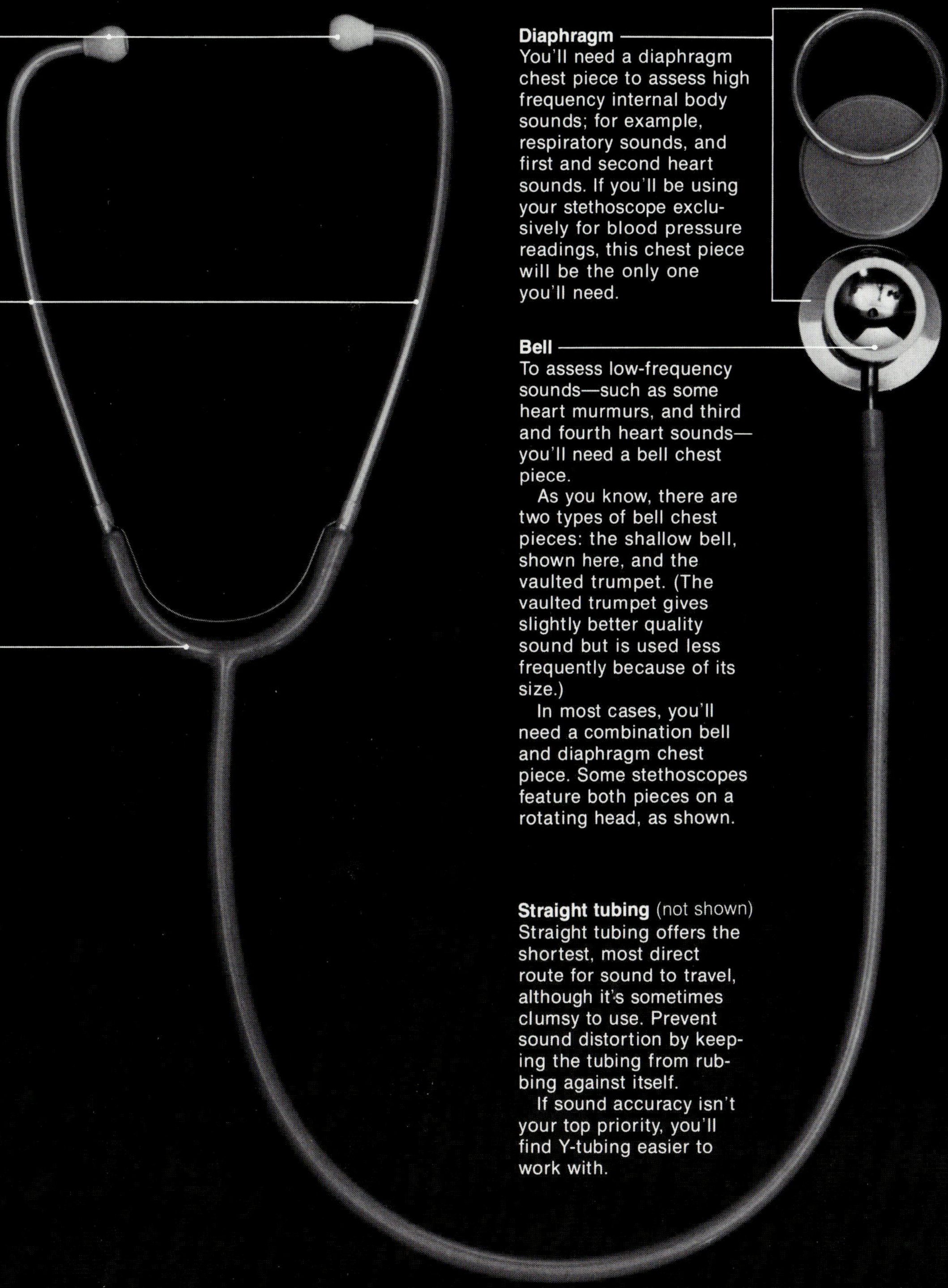

Eartips
Eartips are usually made of hard molded plastic or flexible rubber. Select eartips that fit snugly and comfortably in your ears.

Binaurals
Binaurals have an internal spring or metal bar between them. The bar or spring provides tension to hold the stethoscope snugly in your ears, and also helps to keep the tubing from kinking.

Y-tubing
For accurate sounds, make sure your stethoscope has tubing between 12" to 15" (30.5 to 38 cm) long and ⅜" (3 mm) in diameter. However, longer tubing's OK if you'll be using your stethoscope only for blood pressure readings. Remember, the longer the tubing, the greater the chance for sound loss or distortion.
  Most stethoscope tubing is made from rubber or plastic, as shown here. Although plastic is considered to be durable, rubber is the best insulator.

Diaphragm
You'll need a diaphragm chest piece to assess high frequency internal body sounds; for example, respiratory sounds, and first and second heart sounds. If you'll be using your stethoscope exclusively for blood pressure readings, this chest piece will be the only one you'll need.

Bell
To assess low-frequency sounds—such as some heart murmurs, and third and fourth heart sounds—you'll need a bell chest piece.
  As you know, there are two types of bell chest pieces: the shallow bell, shown here, and the vaulted trumpet. (The vaulted trumpet gives slightly better quality sound but is used less frequently because of its size.)
  In most cases, you'll need a combination bell and diaphragm chest piece. Some stethoscopes feature both pieces on a rotating head, as shown.

Straight tubing (not shown)
Straight tubing offers the shortest, most direct route for sound to travel, although it's sometimes clumsy to use. Prevent sound distortion by keeping the tubing from rubbing against itself.
  If sound accuracy isn't your top priority, you'll find Y-tubing easier to work with.

Respiratory system

Auscultating lung fields

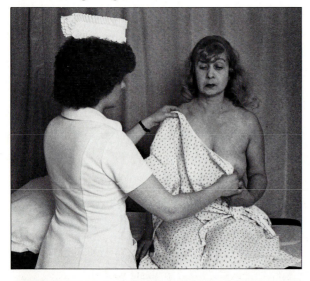

1 *When you auscultate your patient's lungs you're listening for sounds that may alert you to lung abnormalities. To do this effectively, use a stethoscope. Here's how to use it.*

(For information on selecting a stethoscope, see page 77.)

First, seat your patient on a bed or on an exam table (with her feet dangling over the side).

If your patient can't sit up, ask her to lie on her side. However, remember that a side-lying position will decrease your patient's lung excursion. So, when you auscultate and compare both sides of her chest, expect a slightly diminished air flow in her lower lung.

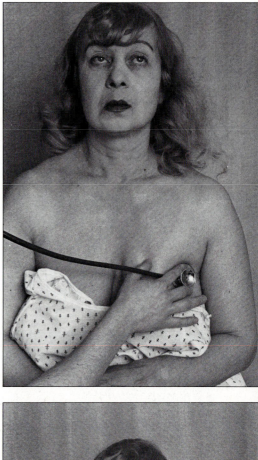

2 Auscultate over your patient's trachea, then down over the bronchi located between her clavicles and midsternum. When you reach the main bronchus, the sounds you'll hear will be loud, high-pitched, and longer on expiration than inspiration. *Note:* If you hear bronchial breath sounds in the *peripheral* lung area, suspect consolidation or atelectasis.

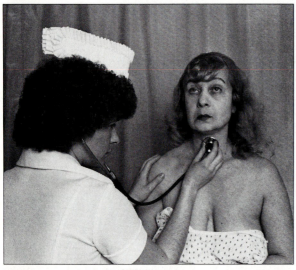

3 Now, auscultate your patient's anterior chest. Follow the sequence used for percussion, on pages 75 and 76.

Expect to hear blowing, bronchovesicular sounds as you auscultate in these areas: over your patient's large airways, on either side of her sternum, at the Angle of Louis, and between her scapulae.

You'll also hear vesicular sounds over the peripheral lung area. These sounds should have a soft, breezy quality.

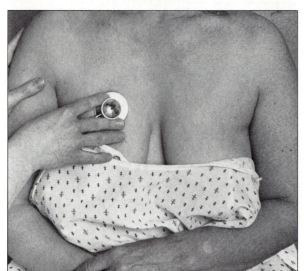

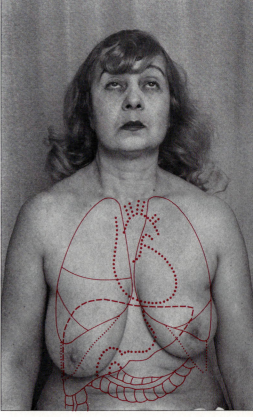

4 As you auscultate, listen for decreased breath sounds, which are fainter and more distant than normal breath sounds. If you hear decreased breath sounds, suspect lung consolidation. Also, listen for the absence of breath sounds, which may mean pneumothorax.

Rales (an intermittent crackling sound) may mean your patient has pneumonia or congestive heart failure.

Do you hear rhonchi (continuous coarse sounds) as you auscultate her large airways? Your patient may have a partial airway obstruction. Instruct her to cough. By coughing, she may clear her airways and enable you to hear other breath sounds.

5 Suppose you detect an abnormality in your patient's lungs? Try to identify its location. To do this, determine the approximate location of your patient's lungs in relation to her chest surface (study this illustration). Document your observations, indicating the lobe or lobes you suspect are affected.

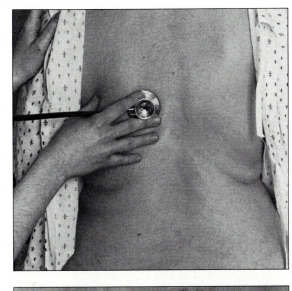

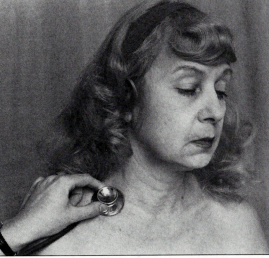

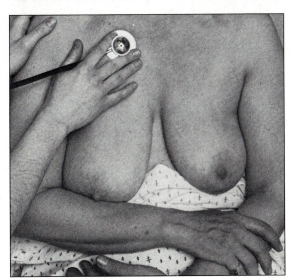

6 Next, auscultate your patient's posterior chest, noting any adventitious (abnormal) sounds.

Nursing tip: If you have trouble identifying normal respiratory sounds, practice listening to your own lungs (provided they're normal).

7 Now, auscultate your patient's anterior chest for vocal fremitus (the sounds produced by your patient's chest vibrations as she speaks). To do this, place your stethoscope's diaphragm slightly above your patient's clavicle.

Then, ask her to repeat "ninety-nine" in her normal speaking voice. As she does, compare the sounds you hear on both sides of her chest. If all's well, you'll hear her voice, but her words will be indistinct. Continue to auscultate your patient's entire anterior chest in this manner.

8 Next, auscultate your patient's anterior chest as she whispers "ninety-nine." As you listen, you'll hear her voice, but her words will be indistinct. Repeat the procedure over your patient's entire anterior chest.

Finally, ask your patient to say "eee." As you auscultate both sides of her chest, you should hear her voice clearly transmitted as "eee."

Repeat these steps for auscultating fremitus on your patient's posterior chest. For more information on evaluating voice sounds, see the NURSING PHOTOBOOK *Providing Respiratory Care.*

Be sure to document your findings.

Respiratory system

Recognizing respiratory patterns

As you're counting your patient's respiratory rate, note her respiratory pattern. Except for an occasional deep breath—is her breathing rhythmical? If her breathing isn't rhythmical, note its depth, rate, and pattern for several minutes. Then document your findings.

This chart will help you recognize the nine major respiratory patterns.

Respiratory pattern	How to recognize it
Eupnea	Normal respiration rate and rhythm. For adults: 15 to 17 breaths per minute; teenagers: 12 to 20 breaths per minute; 2 to 12 years: 20 to 30 breaths per minute; newborns: 30 to 50 breaths per minute. Occasional deep breaths at a rate of two to three per minute.
Tachypnea	Increased respirations, as seen in fever, pneumonia, compensatory respiratory alkalosis, respiratory insufficiency, lesions in the brain's respiratory control center, and aspirin poisoning.
Bradypnea	Slower but regular respirations. Can occur when the brain's respiratory control center is affected by opiate narcotics, tumor, alcohol, a metabolic disorder, or respiratory decompensation. Normal during sleep.
Apnea	Absence of breathing; may be periodic
Hyperpnea	Deeper respirations; rate normal
Cheyne-Stokes	Respirations gradually become faster and deeper than normal, then slower, over a 30- to 170-second period. Alternating with periods of apnea for 20 to 60 seconds. Causes: increased intracranial pressure, severe congestive heart failure, renal failure, meningitis, and drug overdose
Biot's	Faster and deeper respirations than normal, with abrupt pauses between them. Each breath has same depth. May occur with spinal meningitis or other CNS conditions.
Kussmaul's	Faster and deeper respirations without pauses. In adults: over 20 breaths per minute. Patient's breathing usually sounds labored, with deep breaths that resemble sighs. Can occur from renal failure or metabolic acidosis, particularly diabetic ketoacidosis.
Apneustic	Prolonged, gasping inspiration, followed by extremely short, inefficient expiration. Can occur from lesions in the brain's respiratory center.

Identifying lung problems

Assessment variables

	Pneumonia	Emphysema	Asthma	Pneumothorax	Pleural effusion
Cough	• Hacking • Nonproductive at first but later becomes productive and severe as condition progresses	• Chronic • Hacking	• Infrequent • Nonproductive at first but later becomes very productive as attack worsens	• Nonproductive	• Slight, nonproductive cough sometimes present
Sputum	• Tenacious and colored (in late stages)	• Small amount of clear sputum present.	• Large amounts of tenacious sputum present as condition progresses.	• None	• None
Pain	• Sudden and sharp in chest area • Area aggravated by chest movement	• None	• None (some soreness possible after attack)	• Sudden and sharp in chest area	• Usually none
Breathing	• Increased rate • Decreased excursion on affected side	• Prolonged forced expiration, often through pursed lips • Use of accessory muscles, causing intercostal retraction	• Severe dyspnea with prolonged expiration • Intercostal retraction • Respiratory arrest possible	• Dyspnea • Increased rate • Cessation of normal chest movement on affected side	• Dyspnea
Palpation	• Increased tactile fremitus	• Decreased tactile fremitus	• Decreased or normal tactile fremitus	• Decreased tactile fremitus	• Decreased tactile fremitus
Percussion	• Decreased resonance • Decreased diaphragm movement on affected side	• Resonance or (more commonly) hyper-resonance • Diaphragm movement minimal	• Increased or decreased resonance	• Hyperresonance	• Flat or dull sounds • Decreased diaphragm movement
Auscultation	• Rales • Rhonchi	• Decreased or absent breath sounds • Wheezing and rhonchi	• Decreased breath sounds • Wheezing more pronounced on expiration	• Decreased or absent breath sounds over affected side	• Decreased or absent breath sounds over involved area • Egophony and whispered pectoriloquy above fluid level.
Special	• High fever and chills commonly accompany condition.	• Patient may have increased anteroposterior diameter (barrel chest).	• Audible wheezing, extreme anxiety, and perspiration commonly accompany attack.	• Extreme apprehension, restlessness, drop in blood pressure, and rapid thready pulse commonly accompany condition.	• Patient's trachea may shift away from affected side. • Tachycardia present

Cardiovascular system

Do you know how to properly assess your patient's cardiovascular system? Being skilled at palpating, percussing, and auscultating is just part of it. You must also know how to evaluate the results of your examination.

In the next few pages, we'll show you how to:
• determine the size of your patient's heart through percussion.
• grade any heart murmurs she may have.
• identify abnormal heart sounds.

DOCUMENTING

Cardiovascular questions: What to ask
Before you begin assessing your patient's cardiovascular system, you'll want to gather information about your patient's medical history, life style, and family history. Here are some questions to include in your interview:
• Have you ever had any heart problems? If so, have you been treated for them? How? Are you taking any medication for your heart? What is it? How long have you been taking it? How many times a day?
• Has the doctor ever told you that you've had a heart attack? If so, how long ago?
• Have you ever had an electrocardiogram (EKG)? When? Where? Why?
• Do you ever have chest pain? Can you describe it? How long does

Cardiac landmarks: An inside look

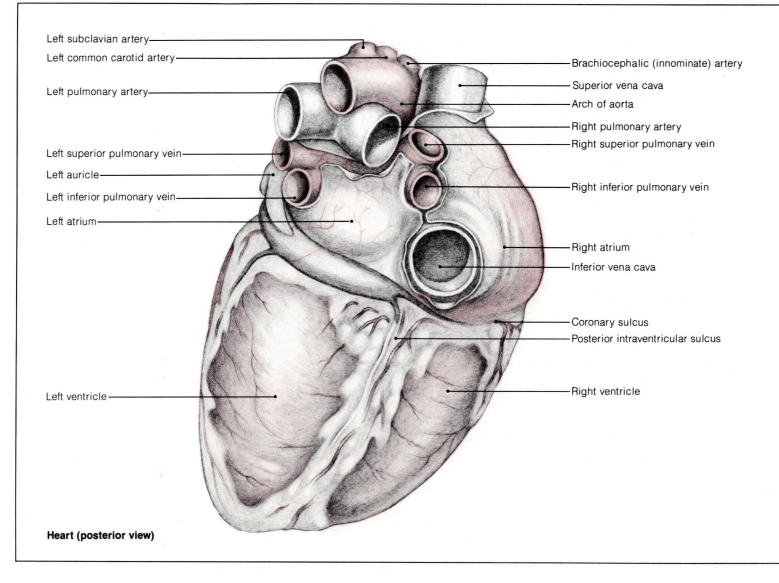

Left subclavian artery

Left common carotid artery

Left pulmonary artery

Left superior pulmonary vein

Left auricle

Left inferior pulmonary vein

Left atrium

Left ventricle

Brachiocephalic (innominate) artery

Superior vena cava

Arch of aorta

Right pulmonary artery

Right superior pulmonary vein

Right inferior pulmonary vein

Right atrium

Inferior vena cava

Coronary sulcus

Posterior intraventricular sulcus

Right ventricle

Heart (posterior view)

it last? Does anything make it worse? Does anything relieve it? Does the pain radiate to your neck? Jaws? Arms? Back? Does the pain ever wake you up at night?
• Do you ever feel like your heart skips a beat? Do you ever feel like it's beating real hard? Do you ever feel flutterings or palpitations in your chest?
• Do you ever experience a shortness of breath? When? Does it wake you up at night? Does it occur after particular activities? Does anything relieve it?
• How many pillows do you sleep on at night?
• Do you have high blood pressure?

• Have any of your relatives had any heart problems? How about high blood pressure?
• Do you smoke cigarettes, a pipe, or cigars? When did you begin smoking? If you no longer smoke, how long ago did you stop?
• Do you drink alcoholic beverages? If so, what type: beer, wine, or whiskey? Do you sometimes have more than one drink a day?
• How often do you exercise? What kind of exercise do you do?
• Do you ever have swollen feet or ankles? Are they swollen when you get up in the morning?
• Are you on any special diets? Do you add salt to your food?
• Can you describe any other problems?

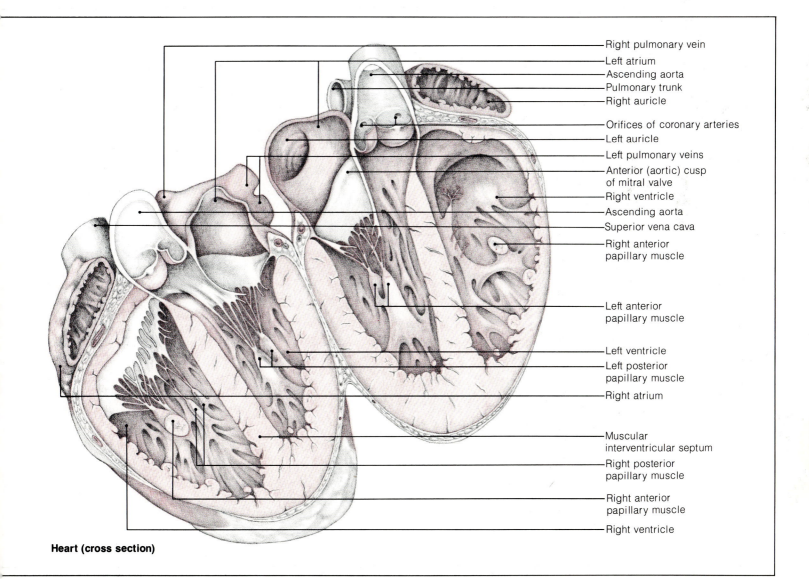

Heart (cross section)

Cardiovascular system

How to assess your patient's heart by inspection and palpation

1 *Now we'll show you how to assess your patient's heart through inspection and palpation. When you do, remember to use the ball of your hand to detect vibrations and thrills. Use your fingertips to identify pulsations.*

Before you begin, make sure the room is warm and private. Explain the examination procedure to your patient and reassure her.

Begin by locating the point of maximal impulse (PMI) at the fifth left intercostal space, medial to the mid-clavicular line. (If you have difficulty locating the PMI, observe your patient's chest, from eye level, as the nurse is doing here.)

In this area, you'll see a slight, well-localized pulsation in the intercostal space. If you see a rib retraction, or pulsation in other areas, suspect cardiac disease.

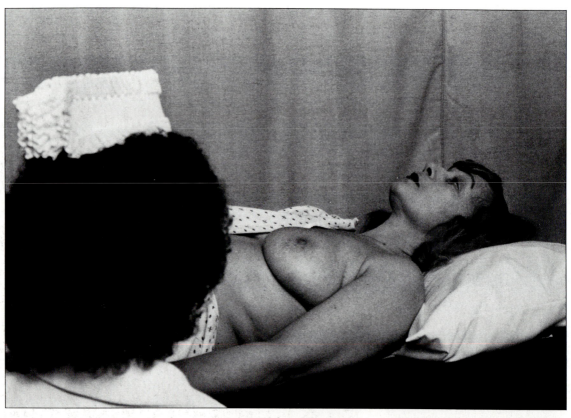

2 Next, use your fingertips and the ball of your hand to palpate for the PMI. Note the beat's amplitude, size, intensity, location, and duration. If all's well, you'll feel a light impulse in an area approximately ½" to ¾" (1 to 2 cm) in diameter.

In most cases, the impulse will begin at the time of the first heart sound, then continue through the first ⅓ to ½ systole. Note any extra impulses.

[Inset] Suppose your patient's overweight or has large breasts. You probably won't be able to see the PMI or palpate it, as explained above. In such a case, ask your patient to roll onto her left side. Then, palpate the PMI's amplitude, size, intensity, and duration, as shown here. Since you turned the patient, you won't be able to document the PMI's location.

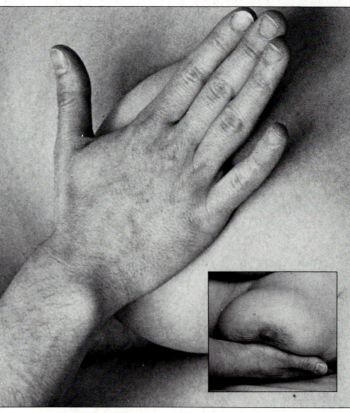

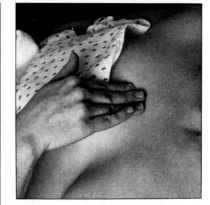

3 Locate the area where the heart's valve sounds are loudest as follows: aortic valve area (second right intercostal space); pulmonic valve area (second and third left intercostal spaces); tricuspid valve area (fifth left intercostal space); and mitral valve area (fifth left intercostal space at the midclavicular line).Then, gently palpate each area with your fingertips and the ball of your hand. Note pulsations and thrills, and feel for the vibration of valve closures.

Palpating your patient's jugular veins, carotid arteries, and peripheral pulses

1 *Suppose you're inspecting your patient's cardiovascular system. Start by examining her jugular veins, carotid arteries, and peripheral pulses. Here's how:*

First, explain the procedure. Then, instruct your patient to lie on her back, with her head slightly elevated (about 15° to 20°). Then, tip her head away from the area you'll be examining.

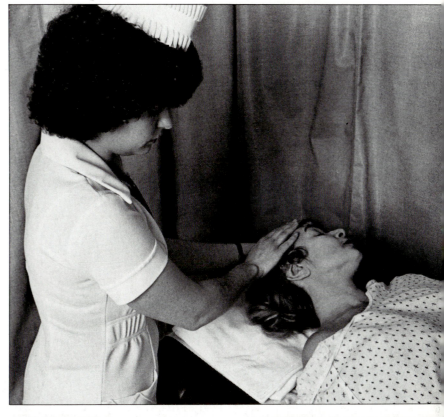

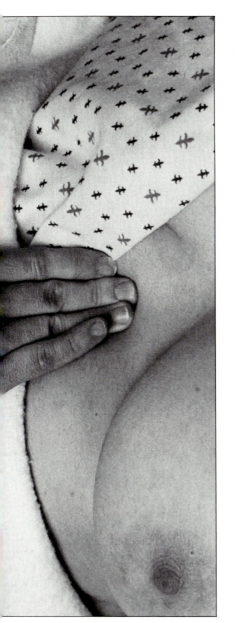

2 Now, locate your patient's right jugular vein, using the illustration on page 87. Gently palpate the vein. If all's well, it'll be pulsating faintly and feel well filled.

However, suppose the vein's distended and pulsating wildly? Notify the doctor at once. Your patient may have elevated central venous pressure.

Repeat the procedure on your patient's left side.

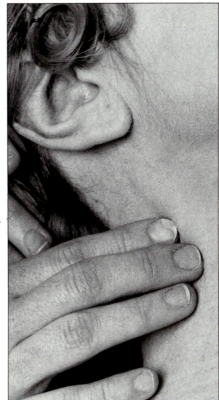

4 Finally, palpate the epigastric area. To do this, slide your fingers up under your patient's rib cage, at the sternum. Hopefully, you'll be able to feel the aorta pulsating against the palmar aspect of your fingertips, and the right ventricle beating against your fingers.

If you feel bounding pulsations, your patient may have an aortic aneurysm.

Remember, if your patient's overweight, you may not be able to feel the abdominal aorta.

Document your findings.

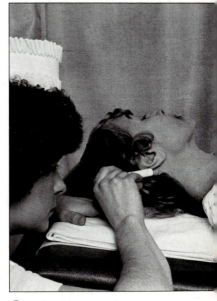

3 What if you can't see any jugular vein pulsations? Shine a flashlight across your patient's lower neck at a tangential angle, as shown here. If everything's OK, you'll see light waves at a rate equal to her arterial pulse.

Cardiovascular system

Palpating your patient's jugular veins, carotid arteries, and peripheral pulses continued

4 Now, strip your patient's right jugular vein. To do this, run your fingers from the base of your patient's neck upward. Then, use one finger to occlude the vein at her jaw level (see inset).

Watch the vein closely; it should fill slowly from its base. If it fills rapidly or pulsates wildly, your patient may have elevated central venous pressure.

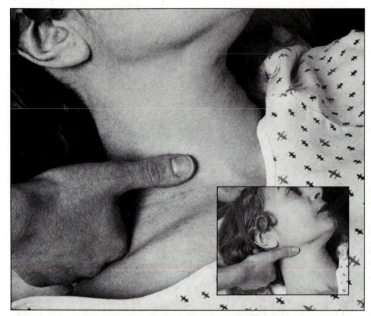

5 Next, slowly raise your patient to a semi-Fowler's position (not greater than 45°). As you do this, observe her right jugular vein. If her venous pressure's OK, the top of the pulsation will be less than 1¼" (3 cm) above the angle where the clavicle and sternum meet. A pulsation *above* this level may indicate elevated central venous pressure.

Observe your patient's left jugular vein in the same way.

🔖 *Nursing tip:* Suppose you *still* don't see a jugular pulsation. Elevate her head higher than 45°. In a patient with extremely elevated central venous pressure, the vein may be so completely filled with blood that pulsations won't be evident.

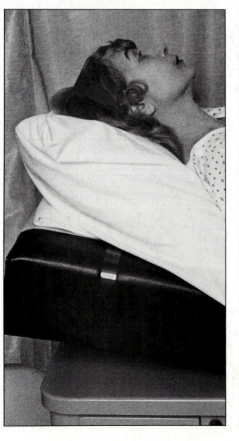

6 Now, locate your patient's right carotid artery, as explained on page 27.

Caution: Avoid pressing on the carotid artery or you may cause bradycardia or asystole.

With your fingertips, count your patient's pulse rate for 30 seconds and multiply by two. Note rate, quality, force, and rhythm.

As you know, an average pulse rate ranges from 60 to 90 beats per minute. If you find any irregularities, count your patient's pulse again; this time for at least a minute. Repeat on your patient's left carotid artery.

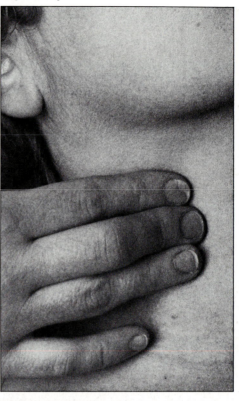

7 Now, check your patient's peripheral pulses. Study the photo on page 87 and locate your patient's brachial pulse. In the same manner explained above, count your patient's pulse for 30 seconds and multiply by two. Note the rate, quality, force, and rhythm.

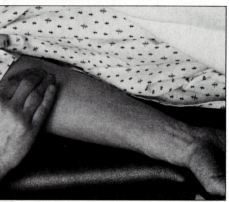

8 Then, check your patient's radial, ulnar, femoral, popliteal, posterior tibial, and dorsalis pedis pulses.

Remember, when you check pulses, always begin with those closest to your patient's heart and move outward.

Finally, document your findings in your nurses' notes.

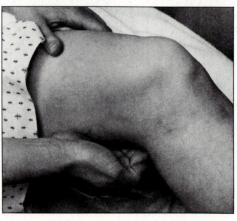

Reviewing the major arteries and veins

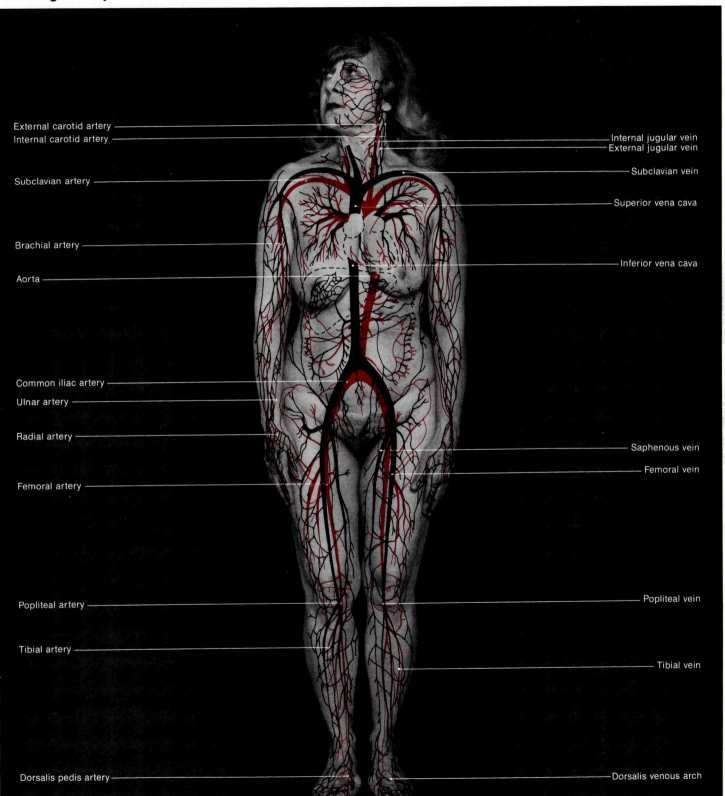

External carotid artery

Internal carotid artery

Subclavian artery

Brachial artery

Aorta

Common iliac artery

Ulnar artery

Radial artery

Femoral artery

Popliteal artery

Tibial artery

Dorsalis pedis artery

Internal jugular vein

External jugular vein

Subclavian vein

Superior vena cava

Inferior vena cava

Saphenous vein

Femoral vein

Popliteal vein

Tibial vein

Dorsalis venous arch

Cardiovascular system

How to perform the Allen's test

1 *Imagine this situation: You're palpating your patient's ulnar artery and don't feel a pulse. Do you know what to do? Use the Allen's test to check the artery's patency. Here's how:*

First, instruct your patient to rest her arm on a desk or table. Support her wrist with a rolled washcloth. Then, ask her to clench her fist.

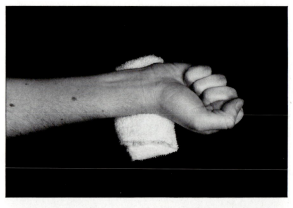

2 Next, using your middle and index fingers of both hands, press on her radial and ulnar arteries, as the nurse is doing here. Maintain the pressure for a few seconds.

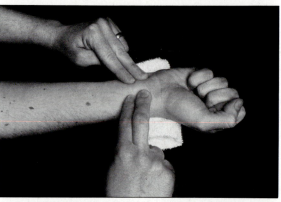

3 Without removing your fingers, tell your patient to unclench her fist, and to hold her hand in a *relaxed* position. When she does, her palm should appear blanched, since you've impaired the normal blood flow with your fingers.

[Inset] Make sure she doesn't *hyperextend* her hand when she unclenches her fist. Doing so would cause false blanching, which would alter the test results.

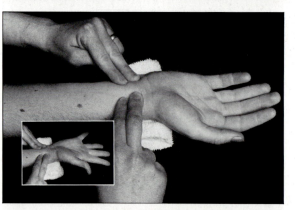

4 Now, release pressure only on your patient's ulnar artery. If the artery's patent, her hand will flush, indicating the rush of oxygenated blood to her hand.

Repeat the test on her other wrist. Then, document your findings in your nurses' notes.

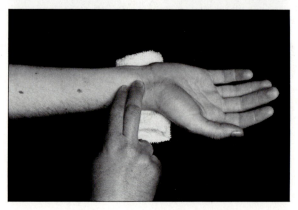

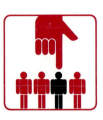

Taking your patient's blood pressure

Are you taking your patient's blood pressure? If so, you'll want to look out for any variables that may affect the reading. To do this, ask yourself these questions:
* Have I chosen the correct size cuff for my patient? (The cuff's bladder should be 20% wider than the diameter of your patient's arm.)
* Have I placed the cuff directly over my patient's brachial artery?
* Is the cuff secure?
* Did I deflate the cuff at the proper rate? (If you deflate it too slowly, you'll get a false high reading caused by venous congestion.)
* Have I taken into consideration that blood pressure rises during the following times: after meals, during (or directly after) exercise, with emotional upset, with a full bladder, or if the patient's arm is below her heart level? (A blood pressure reading will also be slightly higher in a patient's legs.)
* Is my patient lying down, sitting, or standing? (You'll get a slightly lower blood pressure reading if your patient's lying down.)
* Is my patient hypertensive? (If so, take her blood pressure in both arms while she's lying down, sitting, and standing. You shouldn't get more than a 5 mm Hg differentiation in each arm or position.)
* Does my patient have feeble heart sounds? (If so, you may need an ultrasonic doppler to amplify the sounds.)
* Have I checked my equipment lately to make sure it's working properly?
* Finally, have I accurately documented the blood pressure reading? (Remember, a single blood pressure reading is almost always inconclusive. You'll want to know what your patient's *average* blood pressure reading is before you attach significance to one figure.)

How to percuss your patient's heart

1 *As you know, you'll use your percussion skills to locate your patient's left cardiac border. By doing this, you'll be able to tell if her heart's enlarged or displaced. (However, for a more accurate measure of your patient's heart size, compare your findings with your patient's chest X-ray.)*

Here's how to percuss your patient's left cardiac border: First, locate the fourth left intercostal space, as the nurse is doing here.

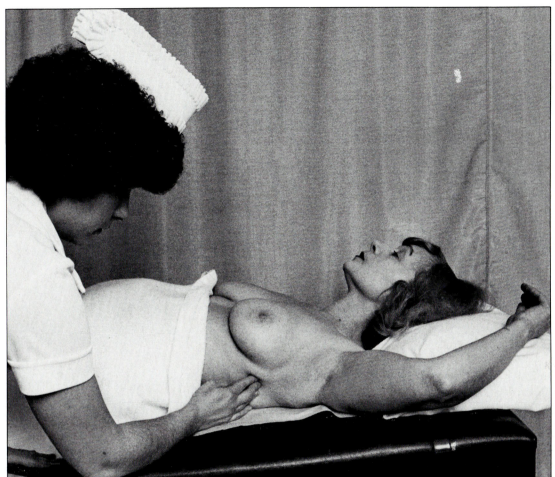

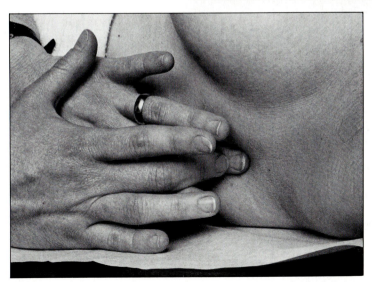

2 Then, place the first joint of your left middle finger parallel to your patient's sternum, between her ribs, on the axillary line.

Now, bring down your striking finger. Expect to hear a resonant sound from the underlying lung. If you don't hear a resonant sound, your patient may have lung congestion.

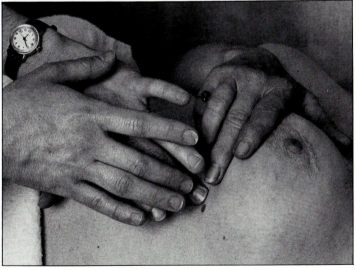

3 Continue percussing along the axillary line, toward your patient's sternum.

When the sound changes from resonant to dull, you've reached the cardiac border. Use a marking pen or stick-on dots to mark the point where you hear the sound change, as the nurse is doing here.

Cardiovascular system

How to percuss your patient's heart continued

4 Now, following the same procedure described in step 3, percuss your patient's fifth and sixth left intercostal spaces. Again, mark the point where the sound changes from resonant to dull.

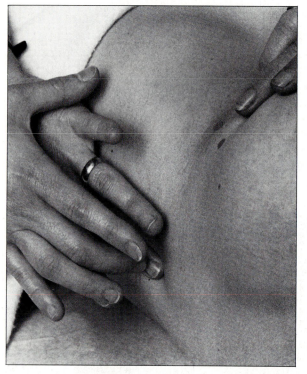

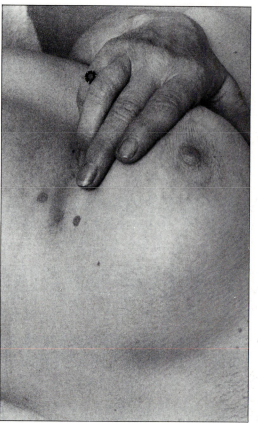

5 Now, mentally connect the points you've marked on your patient's chest; they'll outline the left cardiac border. If you need a more detailed outline of your patient's left cardiac border, percuss along her second and third left intercostal spaces. Mark the points where the sound changes from resonant to dull.

What about the right cardiac border? In most cases, you won't be able to percuss it, because it's directly under your patient's sternum. But you can positively identify her right cardiac border by checking her chest X-ray.

Note: If your patient's obese, you may be unable to percuss her heart. You'll have to check her chest X-ray to identify her heart's size and location.

Finally, document your findings in your nurses' notes.

How to auscultate for your patient's heart

1 *On page 84, we showed you how to assess your patient's cardiac status through palpation. But now, we'll show you how to assess your patient's heart sounds through auscultation.*

Begin by explaining the auscultation procedure to your patient. Then, make sure the room's warm. Instruct your patient to lie flat on her back.

Remove her gown to expose her chest area, and drape her lower body.

Now, warm the stethoscope's bell and diaphragm between your hands, as the nurse is doing here.

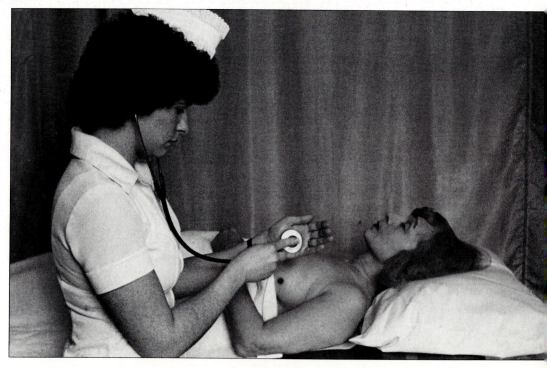

2 Place the stethoscope's diaphragm over your patient's aortic valve area. To locate the correct area, find the second right intercostal space, near the sternal border.

If all's well, you should hear these two normal heart sounds: *lub-dub*, otherwise known as S_1 and S_2. (As you know, the S_1 sound is associated with the closing of the mitral and the tricuspid valves. The S_2 sound is associated with the closing of the aortic and the pulmonic valves.) Note the pitch, intensity, duration, and quality of each sound.

Next, listen for the diastolic and systolic intervals. The diastolic interval is the longer pause between the *dub-lub* (S_2 and S_1). The systolic interval is the pause between the *lub-dub* (S_1 and S_2).

Count your patient's heart beats for a minute, noting rate and rhythm. If you hear an irregular rhythm, describe its irregularity. Is it irregular in a pattern or is it chaotic? If it's a frequent or constant irregularity, notify the doctor. He may want your patient to have an electrocardiogram (EKG).

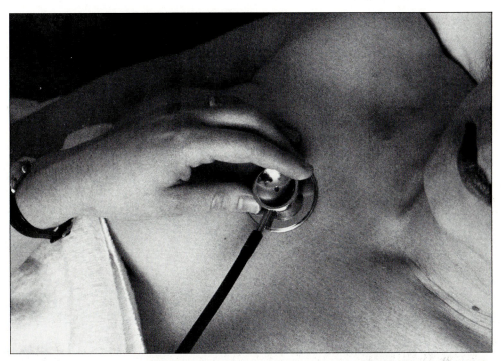

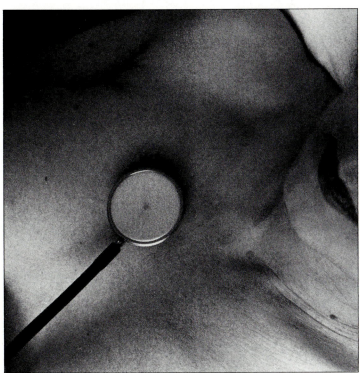

3 Now, lightly place the stethoscope's bell over the aortic valve area. Listen for low-frequency sounds (S_3 and S_4), murmurs, and rubs.

If you have difficulty distinguishing S_3 and S_4, remember their timing in the cardiac cycle. As you know, S_3 occurs *late in the diastolic interval* and S_4 occurs *prior to the systolic interval*. You'll hear S_3 and S_4 louder at the apex.

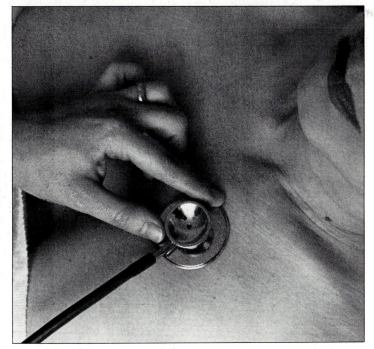

4 Now, use the stethoscope's diaphragm and bell to listen over the pulmonic, tricuspid, and mitral areas. Remember, S_1 sounds louder in the mitral and tricuspid areas, and S_2 sounds louder in the aortic and pulmonic areas. Note the pitch, intensity, duration, and quality of heart sounds in each area. Then, count your patient's heart beat for a minute, noting rate and rhythm.

Also, check for S_3 and S_4 sounds, murmurs, and rubs. (For more information on identifying heart sounds, see page 93.)

Document all findings in your nurses' notes.

Cardiovascular system

Identifying common heart problems

Assessment variables	Mitral stenosis	Mitral regurgitation	Acute myocardial infarction	Congestive heart failure	Acute pericarditis
Palpation	• May feel bounding pulsations to the left of the sternum • Localized diastolic thrill at apex	• Bounding pulsation to left of sternum in late systole • Thrill at cardiac apex during systole	• Abnormal outward movement of precordium or sustained bulge through systole	• Results vary but may include bounding pulsation in left precordium early in diastole	• No characteristic findings
Auscultation sounds	• Loud, snapping first heart sound (S_1) • Rumbling diastolic murmur at heart's apex	• Blowing, high-pitched murmur that occurs throughout systole • Murmur heard at apex, radiating to axilla and posterior chest	• Sounds vary but may include S_3 and S_4, systolic murmurs that are loudest at apex, and pericardial friction rub	• Sounds vary but may include S_3 (early in diastole) and S_2 (split on expiration).	• High-pitched friction rub at left middle and lower sternal border
Pulse	• Weak • Atrial fibrillation (common)	• Usually normal with adequate volume • Atrial fibrillation possible	• Weak • Tachycardia or bradycardia	• Tachycardia	• Normal rhythm • Atrial arrhythmias if condition's severe or prolonged
Breathing	• Dyspnea	• Dyspnea on exertion	• Dyspnea may occur with varying intensity.	• Dyspnea • Orthopnea	• Dyspnea • Tachypnea • Shallow
Pain	• Rare	• Rare	• Usually severe, prolonged chest pain (crushing sensation) • Pain may radiate to neck, back, one or both arms.	• None	• Mild-to-severe substernal pain • Increasing pain on or during inspiration and movement (may radiate to upper arms and back)
Edema	• Peripheral edema • Ascites possible (late stages)	• As condition worsens, peripheral edema possible.	• None (unless caused by complications)	• Peripheral edema (from right-sided heart failure) • Ascites possible	• Possible (if complications present)
Cyanosis	• Common	• Possible	• Frequent	• Common	• Possible
Special	• Patient easily fatigued. • Hemoptysis	• Associated signs and symptoms vary but may include extreme fatigue and reddened cheeks. • Patient may be asymptomatic.	• Nausea • Diaphoresis • Anxiety • Hypotension	• Rales and wheezing • Fatigue • Anorexia, vomiting • Distended jugular veins • Possible enlarged liver and spleen	• Associated signs and symptoms vary, depending on condition's cause. • Joint discomfort and dermatitis possible. • Fatigue • Fever

How to grade heart murmurs

Let's assume your patient has a heart murmur, which you've identified by its timing in the cardiac cycle. Remember to document the murmur's location, quality, pitch, and interval of occurrence.

☎ *Nursing tip:* Wondering how to differentiate a systolic from a diastolic murmur? Palpate your patient's radial pulse as you auscultate for her heart sounds. If the murmur occurs at the same time as her pulse, consider it a *systolic* murmur. If it doesn't, consider it a *diastolic* murmur.

You'll want to note where the murmur sounds the loudest, and where the sound radiates. Grade its intensity, using this chart.

Grade 1: On auscultation, murmur is barely audible.
Grade 2: On auscultation, murmur is faint but can be heard without difficulty.
Grade 3: On auscultation, murmur is soft.
Grade 4: On auscultation, murmur is loud, with a thrill.
Grade 5: On auscultation, murmur is loud but can't be heard without a stethoscope.
Grade 6: Murmur can be heard *without* a stethoscope.

For more information on heart murmurs, see the NURSING PHOTO-BOOK *Giving Cardiac Care.*

Identifying heart sounds

Heart sounds can vary. In order to assess them correctly, use the diaphragm on your stethoscope. Do you have trouble distinguishing one heart sound from another or determining where the sound will be loudest? This chart will help you. Study it carefully.

Type of heart sound	Heart area where sound is loudest	Sounds like	Looks like	Possible causes
First and second heart sound (S₁—S₂)	Apex or Mitral valve area	**Lub**-dub *Also described:* **Lub**-dup	S₁ ... S₂	Normal. S₁ associated with simultaneous closing of mitral and tricuspid valves. S₂ is associated with simultaneous closing of aortic and pulmonic valves.
First and second heart sound (S₁—S₂)	Base	Lub-**dub** *Also described:* Lub-**dup**	S₁ ... S₂	See above
Split S₁ (you'll hear a distinct second component to the first heart sound)	Tricuspid valve area	**T-lub**-dub *Also described:* **Thrup**-dup	S₁ (M T) ... S₂ Mitral valve—M Tricuspid valve—T	Associated with asynchronous closure of mitral and tricuspid valves. Sound may be normal or sign of right bundle branch block.
Physiologic splitting of S₂ (splitting changes during inspiration and expiration)	Pulmonic valve area	Lub-**T-dub** (during inspiration) Lub-**dub** (during expiration) *Also described:* Lub-**thrup** (during inspiration) Lub-**dup** (during expiration)	Expiration: S₁ ... S₂ Inspiration: S₁ ... S₂ (A P) Aortic valve—A Pulmonic valve—P	Associated with asynchronous closure of aortic and pulmonic valves during inspiration. This is a normal response.
Fixed splitting of S₂ (splitting remains constant during inspiration and expiration)	Pulmonic valve area	Lub-**T-lub** *Also described:* Lub-**thrup**	S₁ ... S₂ (A P) Aortic valve—A Pulmonic valve—P	Associated with asynchronous closure of aortic and pulmonic valves that remains constant during inspiration and expiration. Sound frequently heard with right ventricular heart failure.
Third heart sound (ventricular gallop) (S₃) heard early in diastole	Mitral valve area	Lub-dup**a**	S₁ ... S₂ S₃	Early rapid filling of the ventricles. Sound may be early sign of congestive heart failure.
Fourth heart sound (atrial gallop) (S₄) heard late in diastole	Mitral valve area	**Ta**-lub-dup	S₄ S₁ ... S₂	Sound related to atrial contraction and frequently occurs in myocardial infarction or ischemia.

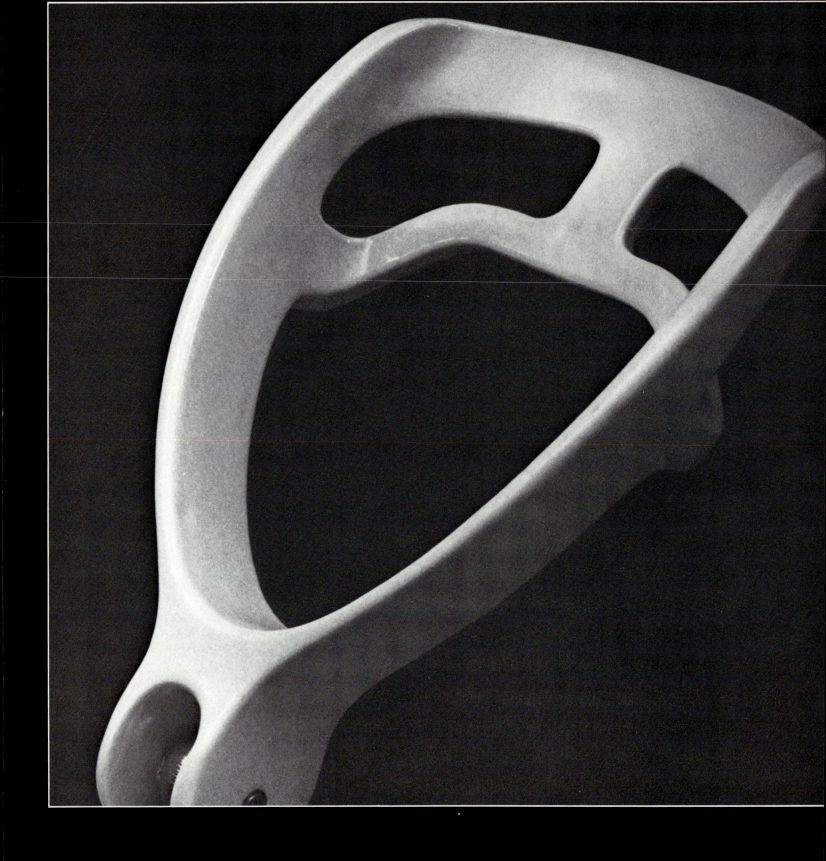

Examining the Abdominal/Pelvic Area

Gastrointestinal system

GU and reproductive systems

Gastrointestinal system

Are you prepared to assess your patient's gastrointestinal system? To do it effectively, you'll need to know how to perform the procedures shown in this section:
• How to observe and inspect your patient's abdomen, as well as document your findings
• How to apply auscultation, palpation, and percussion techniques to abdominal assessment
• How to test your patient for ascites.

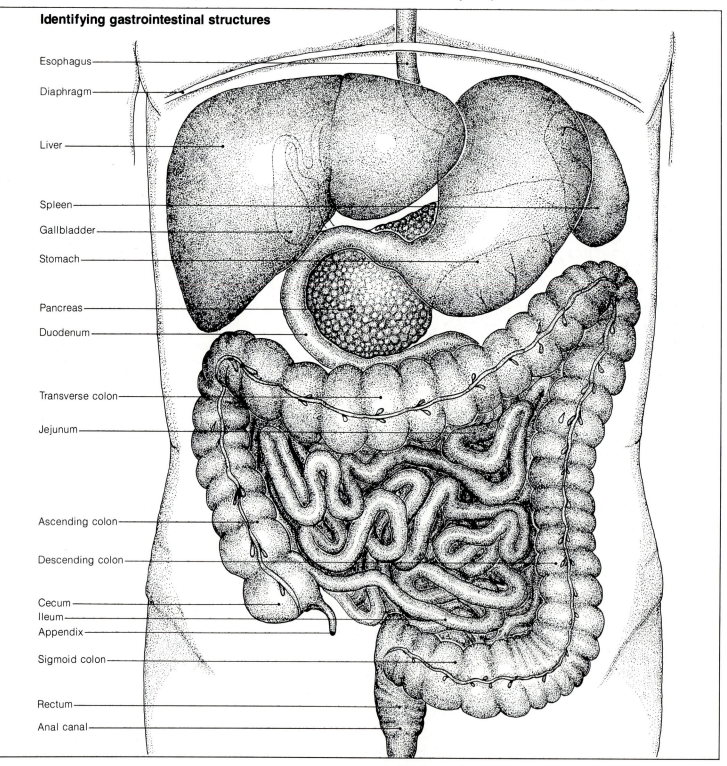

Identifying gastrointestinal structures

- Esophagus
- Diaphragm
- Liver
- Spleen
- Gallbladder
- Stomach
- Pancreas
- Duodenum
- Transverse colon
- Jejunum
- Ascending colon
- Descending colon
- Cecum
- Ileum
- Appendix
- Sigmoid colon
- Rectum
- Anal canal

Inspecting your patient's abdomen

Gastrointestinal questions: What to ask

Assessing your patient's gastrointestinal system? These questions will help you gather the information you need for your data base.

• Have you ever had any pain in your stomach or abdomen? If so, can you describe it? How often do you feel the pain? Is it intermittent, or constant? Does anything relieve the pain or make it worse; for example, eating?
• Do you vomit frequently? If so, describe the vomitus. Have you ever vomited blood? Is your vomitus ever dark brown or black in color? Do you ever take any medication for vomiting? If so, what?
• Have you ever been X-rayed for an ulcer? If so, when? Have you ever been treated for an ulcer? If so, when? Do you still have any pain from your ulcer?
• Have you ever had indigestion, heartburn, or gas? If so, does it usually occur after you eat certain foods? Do you take medication to relieve it? If so, what?
• How often do you have a bowel movement? Do you take laxatives? If so, how frequently? Do you have more than two loose stools a day? If so, do you take medication for this? What kind? Do you ever have blood in your stool? If so, how often? Do you ever have black stools?
• Have you ever had your colon X-rayed? If so, when? Have you ever had a colonoscopy or a proctoscopy? If so, why? How long ago?
• Have you ever had abdominal surgery? If so, when? What type of surgery was it?
• Do you have a colostomy or an ileostomy? If so, how long have you had it? Why was it done? How do you care for it?
• When was the last time you went to a doctor for abdominal or intestinal problems?
• Do you have hemorrhoids?
• Can you describe any other problems?

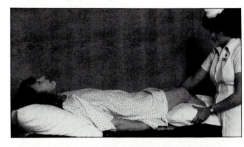

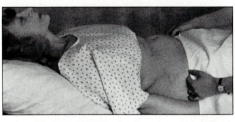

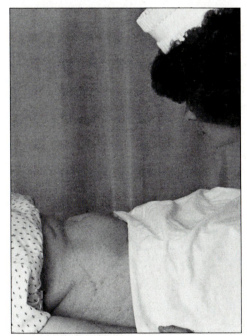

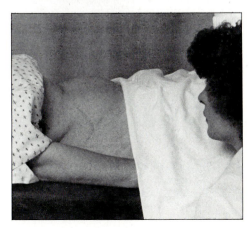

1 *Do you know how to inspect your patient's abdomen correctly? If you're unsure, follow these steps:*

First, instruct your patient to prepare for the examination by emptying her bladder

Now, ask her to lie flat on an exam table in a warm, well-lighted room. To help your patient relax, you may want to place one pillow behind her head and another behind her knees, as shown here.

2 Tell your patient to position her hands at her sides—or on her upper chest—whichever she finds more comfortable.

Then, expose her abdomen from the xiphoid process to the symphysis pubis. Drape the other areas of her body to keep her warm and protect her privacy.

3 Next, inspect your patient's abdomen for overall symmetry. Identify her abdomen's contour as flat, round, protuberant, or scaphoid. If your patient's abdomen appears distended, you may want to test her for ascites (see page 104).

Check your patient's skin for unusual pigmentation, rashes, lesions, hair distribution, and dilated veins. If your patient has striae or abdominal scars from previous trauma or surgery, document their appearance and location in your nurses' notes. (For information on how to document skin abnormalities, see page 21.)

Now, check your patient's abdomen for visible lumps and masses. Check again for possible asymmetry, which may indicate an intra-abdominal mass.

Next, observe the location and contour of your patient's umbilicus. Note any redness, swelling, or umbilical hernia (protrusion of the umbilicus that usually yields to moderate fingertip pressure). Also, look for bluish umbilicus (Cullen's sign), which may indicate intra-abdominal hemorrhage.

4 Now, observe your patient's epigastrium for aortic pulsations. If you can't see the aortic pulsation, look across your patient's abdomen, at eye level.

Note the pulsation's rate, intensity, and location.

Finally, assess your patient's abdomen for peristaltic movement. If all's well, you may either see no movement or a very slight wavelike motion across your patient's abdomen. But if you see undulating waves (especially accompanying a distended abdomen and cramping pain), suspect an intestinal obstruction.

Document all your findings in your nurses' notes.

Gastrointestinal system

How to auscultate your patient's abdomen

1 *Are you auscultating your patient's abdomen? If so, make sure you auscultate before you palpate. Why? Because palpation may change the frequency of your patient's peristaltic sounds. Here's how to auscultate effectively:*

First, picture your patient's abdomen divided into quadrants, as shown here.

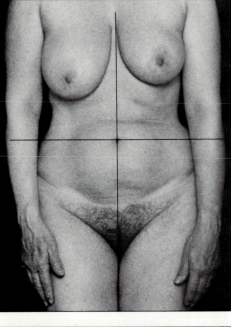

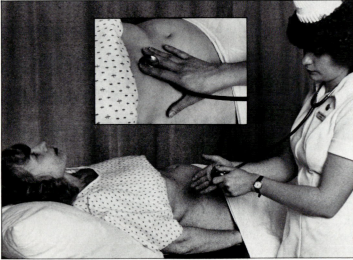

2 Now, warm the stethoscope's diaphragm in your hands, and place it on your patient's upper right quadrant, near her umbilicus (see inset). You should hear intermittent rumbling and gurgling, which are normal bowel sounds.

Count your patient's bowel sounds for 1 minute. If everything's OK, you'll hear 5 to 34 sounds per minute.

If the bowel sounds you hear are loud and occur more frequently than 34 per minute, your patient probably has a hyperperistaltic, nonobstructed bowel.

Carefully listen to your patient's bowel sounds to identify any abnormalities. If you hear frequent, high-pitched, tinkling bowel sounds, or gurgling rushes and loud splashes, your patient may have a bowel obstruction.

Suppose you don't hear any bowel sounds. Continue the procedure, auscultating each quadrant, in clockwise order, for 2 to 5 minutes or until you hear something. If you still don't hear bowel sounds in any of the quadrants, suspect a paralytic ileus.

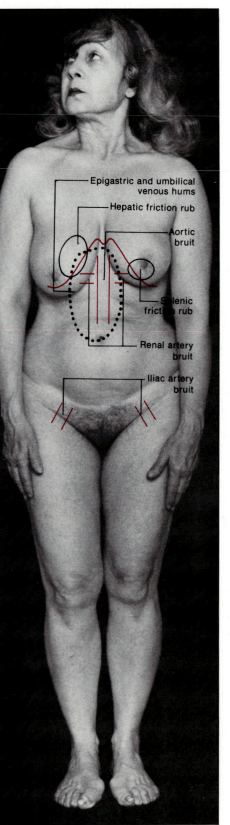

Epigastric and umbilical venous hums

Hepatic friction rub

Aortic bruit

Splenic friction rub

Renal artery bruit

Iliac artery bruit

3 Next, in the areas indicated on this photo, use the stethoscope's bell to auscultate for friction rubs, bruits, or venous hums. Move the bell at 2" to 3" (5 to 7.6 cm) intervals as you auscultate in each area.

As you know, friction rubs sound like two pieces of leather rubbing together. If you hear friction rubs as you auscultate over your patient's liver and spleen, she may have a hepatic tumor or splenic infarct.

You'll recognize bruits when you hear a purring sound. If you hear them in your patient's abdomen, suspect an aneurysm or partial arterial obstruction.

A continuous medium-pitched sound indicates venous hum. If you hear a venous hum when auscultating your patient's abdomen, she may have hepatic cirrhosis.

Palpating and percussing your patient's abdomen

1 *Assessing your patient's abdomen? Here's how to effectively palpate and percuss it.*

First, ask your patient if she has any abdominal pain. If she doesn't, begin percussing any one of her abdominal quadrants, and move in clockwise order. (In this photo, the nurse is beginning with the upper right quadrant.) Remember to keep your finger strikes uniform.

Suppose your patient complains of pain in her upper right abdominal quadrant. Percuss the painful quadrant last.

2 Moving clockwise, percuss all your patient's abdominal quadrants. As you do, mentally note where the percussion sounds change from tympanic to dull. This will help you to identify the location of abdominal organs and detect possible masses.

Do you hear a dull sound in the suprapubic area? Your patient may have a distended bladder.

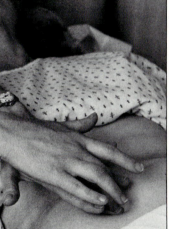

3 Next, *lightly* palpate your patient's abdomen by quadrant, following the same order you used for percussion. Note her skin's temperature. Also, check for tenderness and possible masses. (For more information on light and deep palpation, see page 19.)

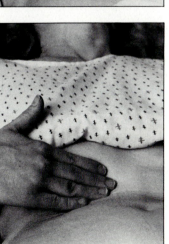

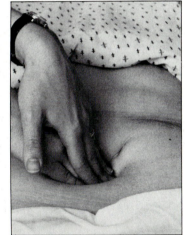

4 Now, *deeply* palpate your patient's abdomen in each quadrant, following the same order as before. Note any organ enlargement, masses, bulgings, or swellings. If you detect a mass in your patient's abdomen, document its location, size, shape, consistency, tenderness, and mobility. Also, note any pulsations you may feel.

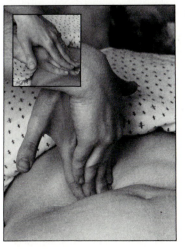

5 Is there a painful or tender area in your patient's abdomen? Check for rebound tenderness, which may indicate peritoneal inflammation.

To detect rebound tenderness, slowly press your fingertips into the tender area.

[Inset] Then, quickly remove them. If your patient complains of sharp pain when you *remove* your fingers, she has rebound tenderness.

Document all your findings in your nurses' notes.

Gastrointestinal system

Assessing your patient's liver

1 *Performing a complete abdominal assessment on your patient? Make sure you properly assess her liver. To learn how, use the guidelines in this photostory.*

Beginning at the level of your patient's umbilicus, percuss upward along her right midclavicular line. Continue until the percussion sounds you hear change from tympanic to dull. The dull sound indicates you've located the lower border of your patient's liver. Mark this location with a marking pen or stick-on dots.

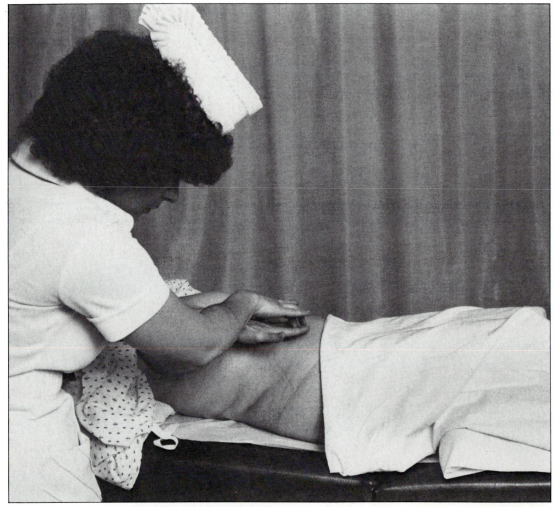

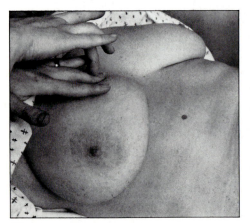

2 Next, locate her right midclavicular line at midsternal level. Percuss downward, along the midclavicular line, until the percussion sounds you hear change from resonant to dull. The dull sound indicates you've reached the upper border of the liver. Mark this location, as before.

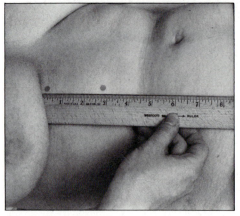

3 Now, measure the distance between the two marks. The distance may be as little as 2⅜" (6 cm) in a small person to as much as 4¾" (12 cm) in a large person. If your patient's liver span measures more than 4¾" (12 cm)—or seems large for her size—she may have an enlarged liver.

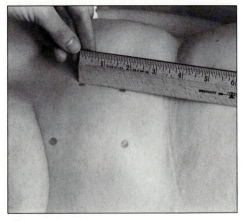

4 Suppose you suspect your patient's liver is enlarged. Repeat the percussion procedure at her midline. The distance between the upper and lower liver borders should be 1¾" to 3¼" (4.4 to 8.2 cm).

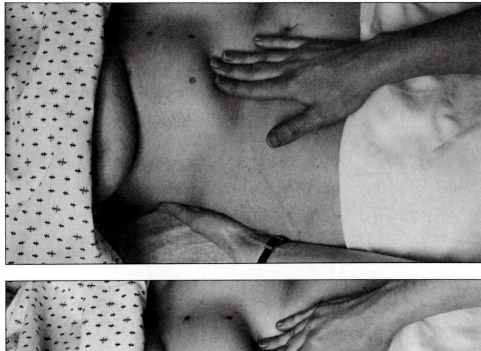

5 Next, use the bimanual technique to deeply palpate the lower edge of your patient's liver. (Remember, the liver's upper portion is located under the rib cage and can't be palpated.)

To palpate the lower edge of your patient's liver, stand at her right side. Place your left hand beneath her back, so her 11th and 12th ribs rest on your palm. Then, place your right hand on her abdomen, so it's parallel to her midline. Make sure your hand is below the stick-on dots indicating the liver's lower border.

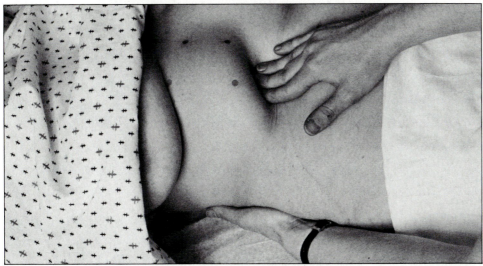

6 Now, instruct your patient to breathe deeply through her mouth. As she exhales, gently press *upward* with your left fingers and *downward* with your right. Try to press a little deeper with each exhalation, until you feel the lower edge of your patient's liver.

You should feel a sharp, firm, regular ridge as the liver's edge meets your fingers. However, in some cases, you may only feel an increased resistance against your fingertips, indicating the liver's lower edge.

If you've reached the maximum palpation depth and still can't feel your patient's liver, move your right hand closer to the right costal margin. Now, repeat the palpation procedure until you palpate the liver's lower edge, feel increased resistance, or conclude that the liver is not palpable.

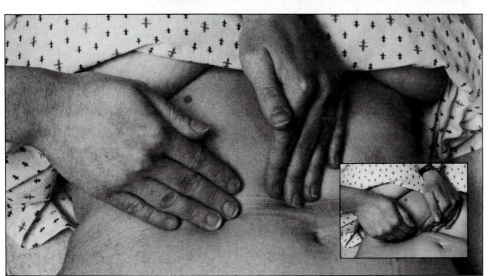

7 You may prefer to use the hooking technique to palpate your patient's liver. To do this, stand at your patient's right side, facing her feet.

Place the fingertips of both your hands on your patient's abdomen, just below the dots indicating the liver's lower border.

[Inset] Now, press down, and gently draw your fingers back toward the right costal margin. Instruct your patient to breathe deeply. As she exhales, you may feel the liver's lower edge or increased resistance.

Document all your findings in your nurses' notes.

Gastrointestinal system

How to assess your patient's stomach and spleen

1 *Now, get ready to percuss your patient's stomach and spleen. First, explain the procedure to your patient. Then, make sure the room's warm. When that's done, proceed as follows:*

Begin percussing slightly above and to the right of your patient's umbilicus. Percuss across her abdomen to her left anterior axillary line. As you do, note where the percussion sound changes from dull to tympanic. (Tympany indicates you're percussing over the stomach.)

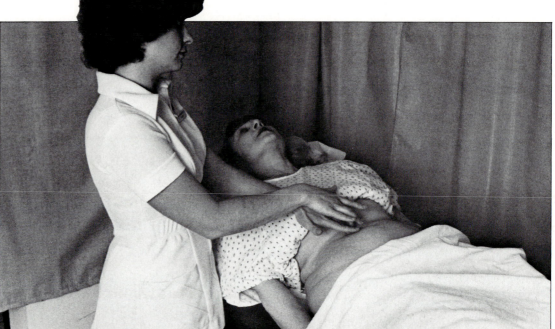

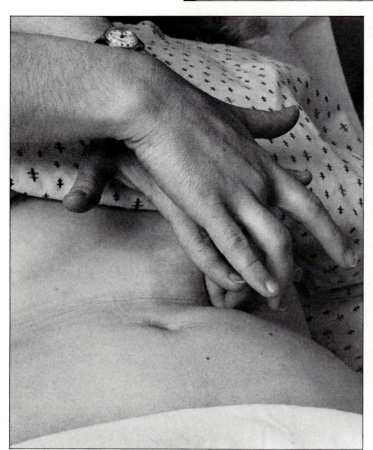

2 Now, percuss across your patient's abdomen about 2" (5 cm) above your first line of percussion. Mentally note where the percussion sound changes, and compare this to your first percussion line.

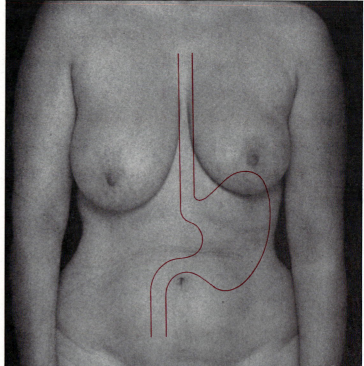

3 Continue the procedure until you've percussed your patient's entire stomach and know its approximate size and position.

This illustration shows a normal stomach and its relative size and location in the abdomen. But remember, the size of your patient's stomach can vary greatly within the normal range.

However, suppose you discover that more than five sixths of your patient's stomach is left of the median line. Suspect an abnormally enlarged stomach, particularly if she also has upper abdominal distention.

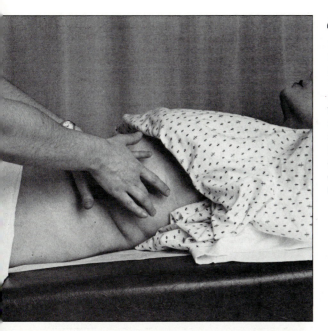

4 To percuss the spleen, locate the area just under your patient's left midaxillary line. Beginning above the 12th rib (at the 11th intercostal space), percuss each interspace up to the 8th rib (7th intercostal space). If your patient's spleen is normal, you should hear tympany as you percuss. But if her spleen's enlarged, you may hear dullness.

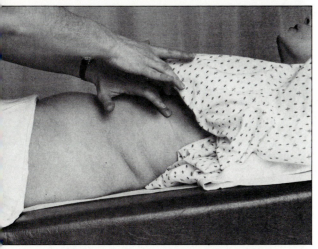

5 If you haven't detected splenic enlargement with this method, locate and percuss along your patient's ninth intercostal space in the anterior axillary line. As you percuss the interspace, you should hear tympany.

Now, ask your patient to inhale deeply, and percuss the same area. If the percussion sound changes from tympanic to dull as your patient inhales, she may have an enlarged spleen.

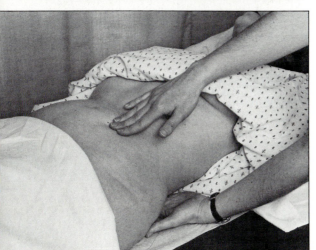

6 Next, palpate your patient's spleen. To do this, use your left hand to support your patient's lower left rib cage, as shown in this photo. Then, gently press the fingers of your right hand under your patient's lower left costal margin.

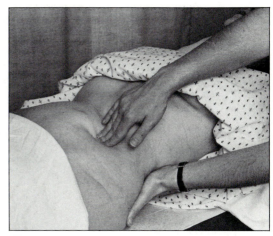

7 Ask your patient to inhale deeply. As she does, lift up with your left hand and press down with your right. If you feel the spleen's edge, the spleen's enlarged to approximately three times its normal size. Note its shape and consistency.

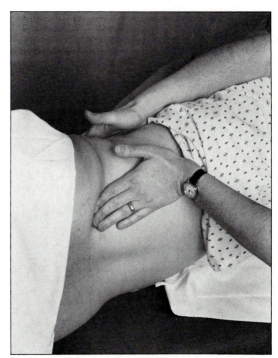

8 If you can't feel your patient's spleen when she's supine, ask her to roll onto her right side. Instruct her to draw her knees up slightly toward her chest. Then, repeat the palpation procedure.

Document any existing splenic enlargement as slight, moderate, or great. Enlargement of ½" to 1¾" (1.3 to 4.4 cm) below the costal margin is considered slight. Moderate enlargement is 1¾" to 3¼" (4.4 to 8.2 cm). Enlargement of 3¼" (8.2 cm) or more is classified as great.

Gastrointestinal system

Palpating the abdominal aorta

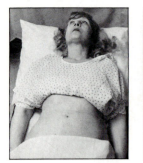 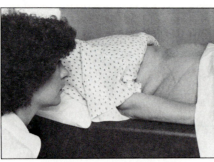 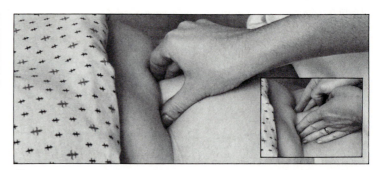

1 *Follow these guidelines carefully to effectively evaluate your patient's abdominal aorta.*

First, locate and observe the aortic pulsation in the epigastric area (slightly to the left of the midline).

2 If you have difficulty locating the pulsation, try looking across your patient's abdomen, at eye level, as shown in this photo.

Then, note the pulsation's rate, intensity, and location. If everything's OK, the pulsation will be faint or absent.

Suppose you see a bounding pulsation. Suspect an aneurysm, and notify the doctor immediately.

3 Next, press deeply but gently into your patient's abdomen, just above the umbilicus. As you do, try to *capture* your patient's aorta between your thumb and fingers.

[Inset] If your patient's abdominal wall is thick, position the fingers of both your hands on opposite sides of the aorta. Then, press down, and try to capture the aorta, as before.

If you're successful, note the aorta's thickness and pulsation. It should be approximately 1¼" (2.7 cm) wide, and the pulsation should exert an upward force against your fingers.

If your patient's aorta is wider than normal, and the pulsations seem to travel from side to side, she may have an aortic aneurysm. Notify the doctor immediately.

Finally, document your findings in your nurses' notes.

Testing for ascites

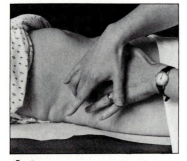 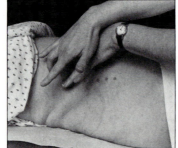 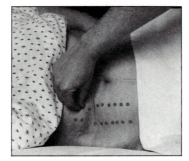 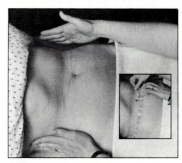

1 *Suppose your patient has a distended abdomen and disproportionately bulging flanks. She may have ascites. Check her abdomen for these other signs: tight, glistening abdominal skin; prominent veins; and umbilical protrusion. If any or all of these signs are present, use the following guidelines to confirm and evaluate her condition:*

First, percuss your patient's right flank. Begin at the iliac crest, on the lowest exposed portion of her flank. Percuss across the flank to her lower rib. If fluid is present in your patient's abdomen, you'll hear a dull sound as you percuss.

2 Return to the iliac crest, and percuss across your patient's right flank, about 2" (5 cm) above your first line of percussion. Repeat this step until you no longer hear dullness. Mark this location with a marking pen or stick-on dots.

Then, percuss your patient's *left* flank, following the same procedure.

3 Now, ask your patient to roll onto her right side. Percuss her abdomen from her right flank upward, toward her umbilicus. Locate and mark the spot where you no longer hear dullness. If your patient has ascites, its border will probably be near her midline.

4 Does your patient have a grossly distended abdomen? Perform the fluid wave test. To produce a fluid wave, place the palm of your hand against your patient's right flank. Now, sharply tap her left flank with your other hand. If your patient has a large accumulation of fluid in her abdomen (advanced ascites), a fluid wave will ripple across her abdomen and cause her right flank to impact against your hand.

[Inset] Finally, measure and record your patient's abdominal girth. Then, if possible, measure her abdominal girth daily, noting any changes.

Document all your findings in your nurses' notes.

DANGER SIGNS

Identifying gastrointestinal problems

Assessment variables	Appendicitis	Acute diverticulitis	Perforated peptic ulcer	Small bowel obstruction	Laennec's cirrhosis
Pain	• Pain pattern varies but may include cramping pain in umbilical area, which may become increasingly intense and localized in lower right abdominal quadrant.	• Constant lower abdominal pain, becoming increasingly severe • Possible abdominal cramping	• Sudden, severe upper abdominal pain, beginning in epigastrium and spreading over abdomen. May radiate to top of right shoulder.	• Intermittent, severe colicky pain, usually in the umbilical area	• Some discomfort present
Nausea/ vomiting	• Both possible after onset of pain	• Nausea common; vomiting rare	• Both possible	• Vomiting soon after onset of pain • In later stages, vomitus has foul, fecal odor.	• Nausea may occur. • Severe hematemesis occurs if esophageal varices rupture.
Elimination problems	• Mild constipation	• Bowel movements become fewer or cease altogether during acute attack.	• No bowel sounds or bowel movement	• Complete obstruction may keep patient from passing flatus or stool. • Incomplete obstruction may cause intermittent diarrhea.	• Chronic constipation
Percussion	• No characteristic findings, unless complications develop	• No characteristic findings	• If air accumulates in peritoneal cavity, liver area may sound tympanic.	• Air-filled bowels sound tympanic.	• Shifting dullness or fluid wave may indicate ascites. • Liver enlargement common.
Palpation	• Rebound tenderness in lower right quadrant, midway between umbilicus and right iliac crest • Muscular guarding	• Local and rebound tenderness may be present in lower left abdominal quadrant. • Mass may be felt in left iliac fossa. • Muscular guarding as condition worsens	• Abdomen tender • Abdomen has boardlike rigidity.	• Abdomen soft at first, then distended and tender. • Muscular guarding and rebound tenderness	• Liver size may vary. • Liver feels firm, with sharp edge. • Enlarged spleen may occur with portal hypertension.
Auscultation	• No characteristic findings	• Hypoactive bowel sounds	• Bowel sounds absent	• Rushes of high-pitched, loud bowel sounds (above obstruction) • Absence of bowel sounds indicates serious complications.	• No characteristic findings
Special	• Anorexia • Low-grade fever	• Moderate temperature elevation may occur. • Anorexia	• Pallor and profuse diaphoresis in condition's early stages • Splinting, accompanied by rapid, shallow breathing • Shock, developing rapidly	• Asymmetrical abdominal distention may occur in late stages of condition. • Dehydration • Peristalsis may be visible above obstruction.	Associated symptoms vary but may include: • Anorexia, fatigue, and weight loss in condition's early stages • Testicular atrophy and enlarged breasts in men • Amenorrhea in women • Palmar erythema, prominent abdominal wall veins, mild jaundice, ascites, ankle edema, and finger clubbing; also, possible massive gastrointestinal hemorrhage

GU and reproductive systems

Reviewing male reproductive structures

Knowing how to evaluate your patient's genitourinary and reproductive systems is an important part of assessment.

Are you familiar with the techniques and equipment you'll use? Whether your patient is male or female, the photostories, charts, and anatomical illustrations on the following pages will help you prepare.

You'll also find bladder and kidney palpation techniques explained in detail. In addition, you'll find step-by-step information on how to examine your patient's genitals and reproductive organs.

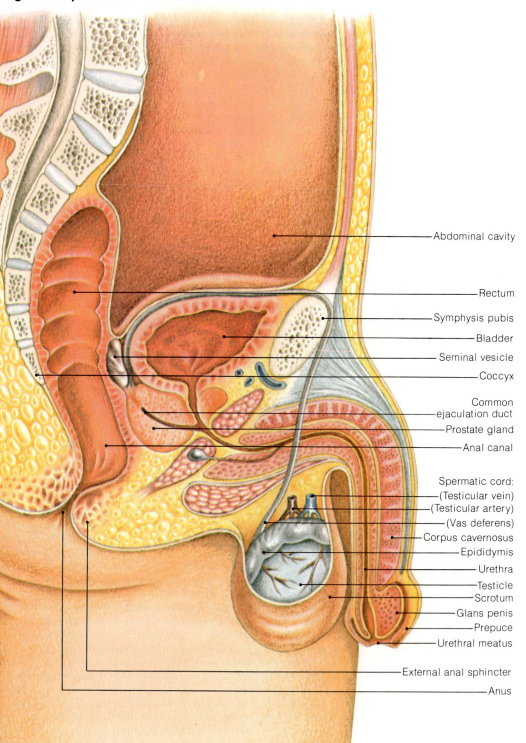

- Abdominal cavity
- Rectum
- Symphysis pubis
- Bladder
- Seminal vesicle
- Coccyx
- Common ejaculation duct
- Prostate gland
- Anal canal
- Spermatic cord:
- (Testicular vein)
- (Testicular artery)
- (Vas deferens)
- Corpus cavernosus
- Epididymis
- Urethra
- Testicle
- Scrotum
- Glans penis
- Prepuce
- Urethral meatus
- External anal sphincter
- Anus

Reviewing female reproductive structures

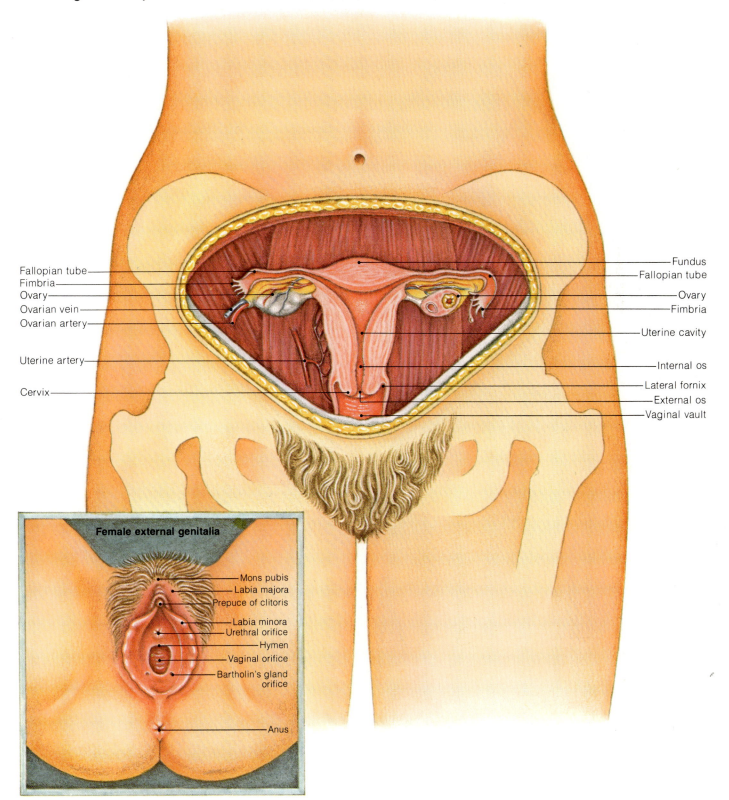

Fallopian tube
Fimbria
Ovary
Ovarian vein
Ovarian artery

Uterine artery

Cervix

Fundus
Fallopian tube
Ovary
Fimbria

Uterine cavity

Internal os

Lateral fornix
External os
Vaginal vault

Female external genitalia

Mons pubis
Labia majora
Prepuce of clitoris
Labia minora
Urethral orifice
Hymen
Vaginal orifice
Bartholin's gland orifice

Anus

GU and reproductive systems

Identifying GU organs, arteries, and veins

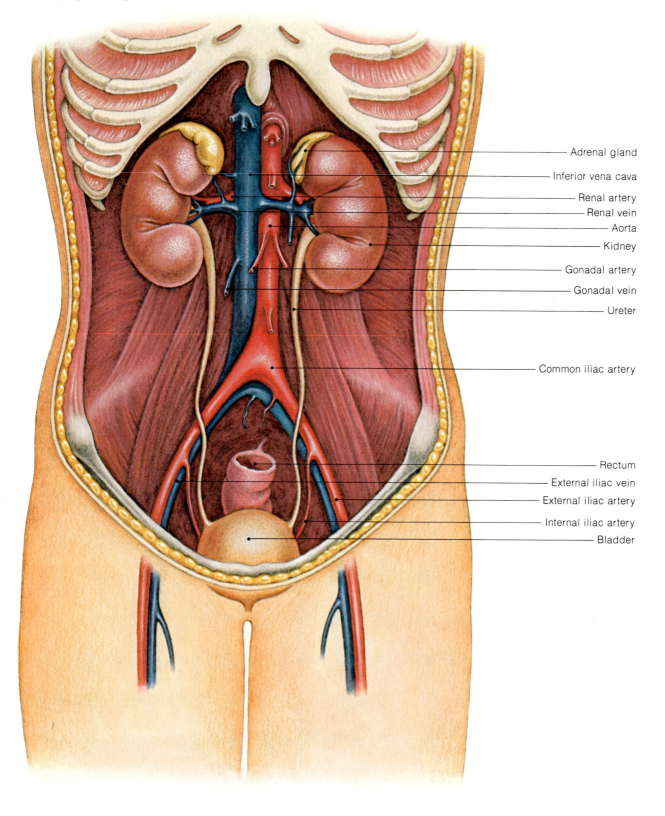

- Adrenal gland
- Inferior vena cava
- Renal artery
- Renal vein
- Aorta
- Kidney
- Gonadal artery
- Gonadal vein
- Ureter
- Common iliac artery
- Rectum
- External iliac vein
- External iliac artery
- Internal iliac artery
- Bladder

GU and reproductive system questions: What to ask

Look over these sample questions for genitourinary and reproductive system assessment. You'll find them helpful in gathering information as you interview your patient. Or use these samples to develop questions of your own.

• How many times a day do you urinate? Have you noticed an increase or decrease in your *frequency* of urination? Have you noticed an increase or decrease in the *amount* of your urine?
• When you urinate, do you ever have trouble starting the flow?
• Has your urine stream changed in size? If so, can you describe it?
• When you're finished urinating, does your bladder feel completely empty?
• Do you wake up at night needing to urinate? How often does this occur? Does it happen only when you drink an unusual amount of fluid before retiring?
• Do you have any problems with your kidneys or bladder? If so, what kind? Have you ever had any kidney or bladder problems; for example, an infection?
• Have you ever had kidney or bladder stones? If so, when? How were they treated?
• Do you ever have a burning sensation when you urinate? If so, how often?
• What color is your urine? Does it ever look red, brown, or black?
• Have you ever had a kidney injury? If so, when? How was it treated?
• Have you ever had surgery on your bladder or kidneys? What kind of surgery did you have? How long ago was it?
• Have you ever had syphilis, gonorrhea, or any other venereal disease? How long ago? How was it treated?

If your patient's a female, consider these additional questions:
• Do you have a problem with leaking urine? If so, does it leak constantly? Does it leak only when you laugh or cough?
• When was your last menstrual period? How often do you get your periods? Are your periods ever irregular? If so, describe the details. How many days do your periods last? Do you ever have pain or cramping with your periods? Does the pain or cramping affect your daily routine? If so, how? Do you have heavy flow with your periods? How many tampons or sanitary napkins do you use in one day? Do you retain water during your periods? Do your hands or feet ever swell? Do you have any

other problems with your periods?
• Are you pregnant now? Have you ever been pregnant? If so, how many times?
• How many children do you have?
• Have you ever miscarried? If so, have you miscarried more than once? When?
• Have you ever had a tubal pregnancy or any other kind of problem pregnancy?
• Have you ever had an abortion? If so, when?
• Have you tried to become pregnant without success? If so, were you tested for fertility problems?
• Is your sexual life satisfying? Is there anything about it you would like to change or improve?
• Do you practice birth control? If so, what method do you use? How long have you been using this method? Is it satisfactory?
• (For a patient who uses birth control pills.) How long have you been on the pill? What type of pill are you taking? Have you ever had any problems that you feel may be associated with taking the pill; for example, headache, localized pain in your calves or chest? If so, describe them.
• Do you ever have any sores or ulcers on your genitals? If so, how often? Are they painful? Do they ooze or drain?
• Do you have any vaginal discharge? If so, describe it. Does any pain or itching accompany it?
• When did you have your last Pap smear? Have you ever had an abnormal Pap smear?
• Have you ever had surgery on your uterus, tubes, or ovaries? Why was it necessary? How long has it been since your surgery?
• Do you have any other problems?

If your patient's a male, consider these additional questions:
• Are you circumcised or uncircumcised?
• (For the uncircumcised patient.) Do you have trouble retracting your foreskin? After it's retracted, can you easily return it to its normal position?
• Have you noticed a change in the skin color of your penis? If so, describe it. Do you have any discharge from your penis? If so, when did you first notice it?
• Are you able to sustain an erection? Have you noticed a change in your sex drive?
• Have you ever had problems with your testes, such as pain or swelling?
• Have you ever been treated for a prostate problem?
• Have you ever had prostate surgery?
• Do you take medication to correct a hormonal imbalance?
• Can you describe any other problems?

GU and reproductive systems

How to examine your patient's external genitalia

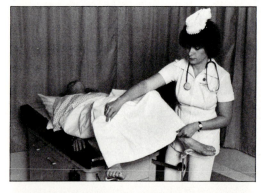

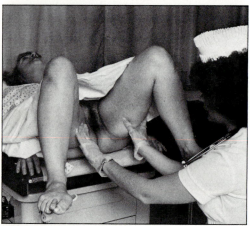

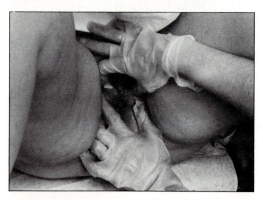

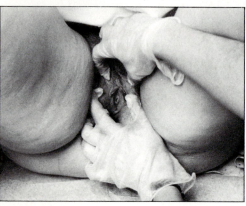

1 *In this photostory, we'll show you how to examine your female patient's external genitalia. (For details on how to examine a male patient's genitalia, see pages 120 through 128.)*

Before you begin, ask your patient to urinate. Then, instruct her to lay on an exam table, with her feet in the stirrups. Drape your patient's thighs and symphysis pubis. Then, ask her to slide forward, so her buttocks are at the table's edge.

Explain the examination procedure to your patient, and make sure the room's well lighted. Then proceed as follows.

2 Slip a pair of clean gloves on your hands. Then, sit on a low stool or chair between your patient's legs.

Observe her pubic hair. Is it excessive? Absent? Sparse? Little or no pubic hair may be caused by advanced age or a hormonal deficiency. Also, check the area for lice.

Next, examine your patient's labia majora and perineum. Expect the labia majora to be slightly prominent and a darker pink than the surrounding tissue. The epithelial surfaces of both structures should be unbroken, symmetrical, and free from masses, fistulae, and abnormal exudate.

Expect the anal opening to be brown and puckered. Note any hemorrhoids, or protruding pink tissue.

3 Now, spread apart your patient's labia majora with your right thumb and index finger. You should see the labia minora, urethral orifice, clitoris, vaginal orifice, and hymen. Each should appear evenly pink. Note any redness or uneven pigmentation.

If you see any lumps, masses, nodules, abnormal exudate, or discharge, document their location, size, and color.

Estimate the size of your patient's clitoris. If the clitoris appears atrophied or is larger than 3/16" (0.5 cm) in diameter, note it carefully.

4 Next, observe the urethral area, noting any redness, discharge, or ulcerations.
Check your patient's vaginal opening. Is it *closed, open,* or *gaping?*

Also, note whether the hymen appears *imperforate, perforate,* or *torn.*

Finally, look near the base of your patient's vaginal opening for her Bartholin's glands openings. If everything's OK, you won't see any. But if you do, note their size and color. Check for possible tenderness, as well as any discharge that may be draining from them. Then, refer your patient to a doctor.

Document all your findings in your notes.

Examining the pelvis and bladder

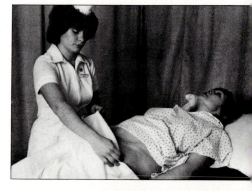

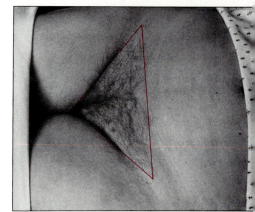

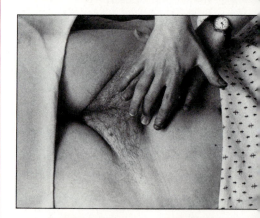

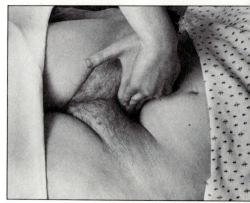

1 *Before you begin examining your patient's bladder and pelvis, ask her to urinate. Explain the procedure, and instruct her to lie flat on an exam table. Then, follow these steps:*

2 First, observe your patient's pelvis, which should be symmetrical and shaped like an inverted triangle. Note any lumps, masses, broken skin, ulcerations, or discolorations.

Inspect your patient's escutcheon. Her pubic hair should begin at the upper edge of her mons pubis and extend downward over her labia. In some women, it forms a diamond-shaped pattern.

Don't consider excessive amounts of pubic hair significant unless your patient also has an excessive amount of body hair.

3 Now you're ready to assess your patient's bladder. Remember, if your patient's a male, you'll follow the same steps.

First, percuss the area over the bladder. If everything's OK, you'll hear a tympanic sound. But if you hear a dull sound, the bladder may be distended from retained urine.

4 Next, locate the *edge* of your patient's bladder. To do this, deeply palpate in her midline about 1" to 2" (2.5 to 5 cm) above her symphysis pubis. Continue to palpate the bladder, noting its size and location. Also note any lumps, masses, or tenderness.

Finally, describe all your findings in your nurses' notes.

Using palpation to assess your patient's kidneys

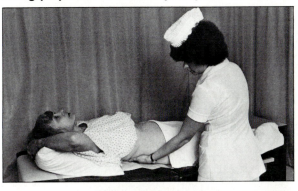

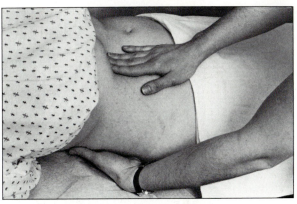

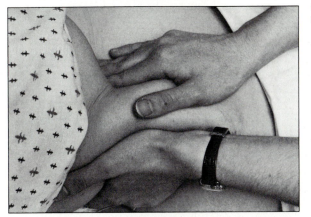

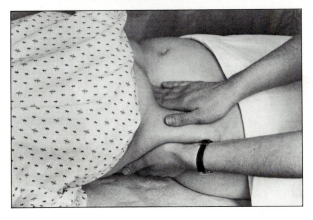

1 *If you're assessing your patient's kidneys by palpation, you'll follow the same steps for both male and female patients.*

First, instruct your patient to lie flat on her back on an exam table. Then, expose her abdomen from her xiphoid process to her symphysis pubis. Stand at your patient's right side.

Now, place your left hand underneath your patient, midway between her lower costal margin and her iliac crest.

2 Position your right hand on your patient's abdomen, directly above your left hand. Angle your right hand slightly toward the costal margin, as shown here.

3 Now, lift up with your left hand as you press down with your right. Each time your patient inhales, press your right hand deeper into her abdomen, until you reach the maximum palpation depth.

Then, tell your patient to inhale deeply. As she does, you should feel the lower pole of her right kidney move down between your hands. Note the kidney's contour and size. Also check for any lumps, masses, or tenderness.

Move your hands to your patient's left side and palpate for her left kidney, using the same method.

4 Suppose you don't feel your patient's kidneys. Try using another palpation technique known as *capturing the kidney*.

To do this, position your hands as you did in step 2. Instruct your patient to inhale deeply. At the peak of her inhalation, quickly—but gently—press your hands together.

GU and reproductive systems

Using palpation to assess your patient's kidneys continued

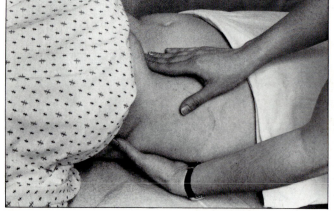

5 Now, tell your patient to exhale as slowly as possible. When she's exhaled completely, slowly release your hands. As you do, you may feel your patient's kidney slide between your hands.

If your patient's kidney is palpable, note its contour and size. Also check for lumps, masses, or tenderness. Mentally note the right kidney's size. It should be about 4¼" (11.4 cm) long, 2" to 3" (5 to 7.6 cm) wide, and 1" (2.5 cm) thick.

Next, move to your patient's left side, and palpate for her left kidney, using the same method as before. Compare the left kidney's contour and size to the right kidney's. But remember, in most cases, your patient's right kidney will be slightly lower than her left kidney. Is one of your patient's kidneys much smaller than the other? Note this carefully; it may be malfunctioning.

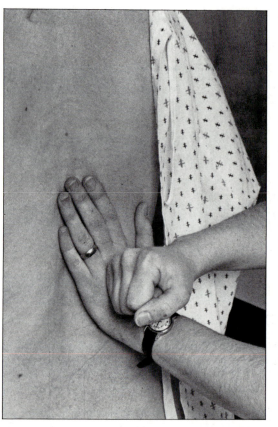

6 Suppose you can't feel your patient's kidneys using either palpation technique. Then, try this method to check her kidneys for tenderness.

Ask your patient to sit up. Place your left palm on your patient's back, slightly to the right of her costovertebral angle. Hit the back of your left hand with your right fist. If your patient feels pain, she may have a kidney infection.

Repeat the procedure on your patient's left side.

Finally, document all your findings in your nurses' notes.

How to use a vaginal speculum

1 *Do you know how to use a vaginal speculum properly? If you're uncertain, follow the guidelines in this photostory.*

First, select an appropriate sized vaginal speculum for your patient.

Note: Small or medium specula are usually best for adolescents and for women who've reached menopause. (The nurse in this photostory is using a medium-sized Welch Allyn prelubricated disposable speculum.)

Hold the speculum's blades under warm running water. This activates the lubricant and warms the blades, making the procedure more comfortable for your patient.

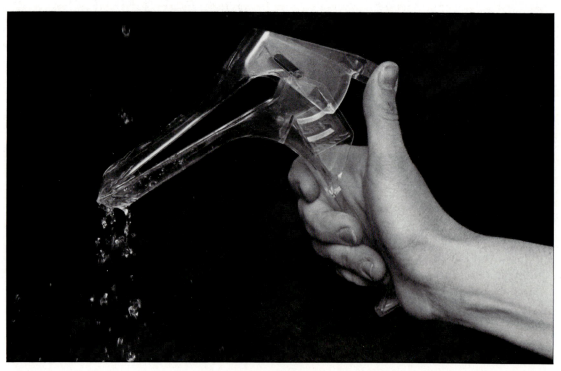

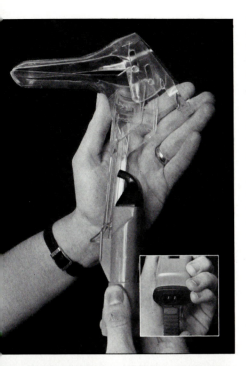

2 Next, attach the vaginal illuminator to the speculum. To do this, hold the illuminator in your right hand. Insert the speculum handle into the channel of the illuminator, as shown here. Push the speculum down the channel until it clicks into place.

[Inset] Then, plug the socket end of the illuminator cord into the bottom of the illuminator handle. Plug the other end into an electrical outlet.

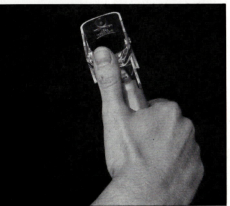

3 Now you're ready to position the speculum for insertion into your patient's vaginal canal. To do this, hold the speculum in your right hand. Rest your thumb on the speculum's lever. With the blades pointing down, tilt the speculum at a 45° angle. (See page 114 for details on how to insert the speculum into your patient's vagina.)

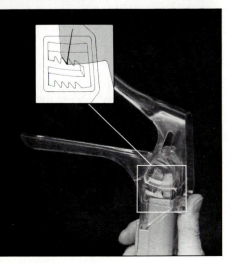

4 When you've inserted the speculum into your patient's vagina, press the thumb lever to open the speculum's blades as far as possible (without causing your patient any discomfort). As you release your thumb, the lever will lock itself in place in one of the notches on the speculum's handle (see inset).

Note: For patients with large vaginas, adjust the thumb lever so it catches the upper tier of notches.

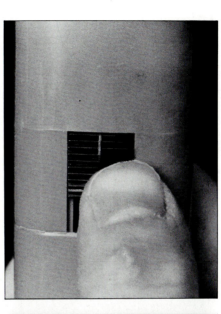

5 Next, switch on the illuminator to light the vaginal canal. Then, do a vaginal exam, as explained earlier.

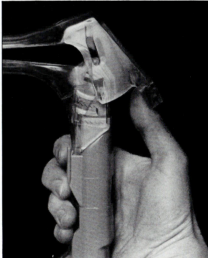

6 When you're finished, press the thumb lever on the speculum up and back to unlock the blades. Close the blades gradually as you withdraw the speculum from your patient's vagina. When the blade tips reach the vaginal opening, close them *completely.* Then, withdraw the speculum, and switch off the illuminator.

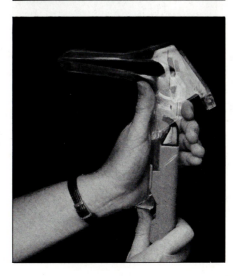

7 Remove the illuminator from the used speculum. To do this, grasp the illuminator in your right hand, and push up on the base of the speculum, being careful not to contaminate your hands.

Finally, dispose of the used speculum.

GU and reproductive systems

How to examine your patient's vagina and cervix

1 *Examining your patient's vagina and cervix? Begin by gathering this equipment: a vaginal speculum with illuminator (or light source), gloves, bifid spatula, normal saline solution (not shown), long cotton swabs, four glass specimen slides, Agar plate, and CytoPrep ™ fixative.*

Slip the gloves on your hands. Then, get ready to insert the speculum into your patient's vagina. Before you do, reassure and relax your patient by gently touching her inner thigh as you explain the exam procedure.

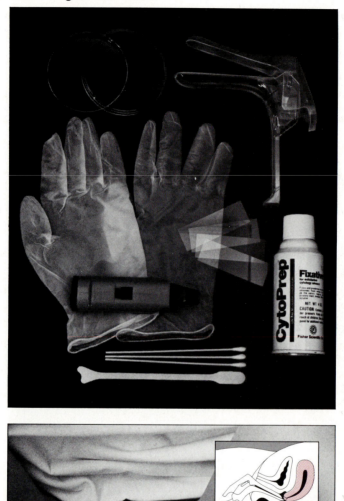

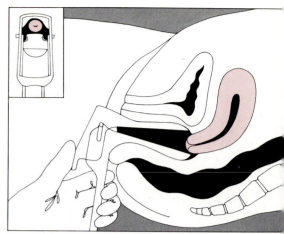

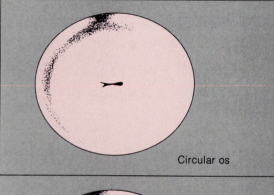

Circular os

Stellate os

2 Now, study this photo. Following the steps on page 113, prepare the vaginal speculum, and position it at a 45° angle, with the blades pointing down.

Spread apart your patient's labia majora, using your left thumb and index finger. Insert the speculum into her vagina.

[Inset] As you do, gently press the speculum against the posterior vaginal wall to avoid irritating the anterior wall and the urethra.

When you've inserted the speculum blades ¼ of the way into the canal, remove your left hand from your patient's labia. Continue to insert the speculum, rotating it to a horizontal position. You should have the speculum handle at a 90° angle to the floor.

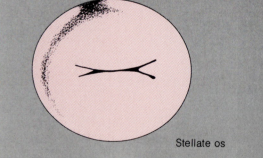

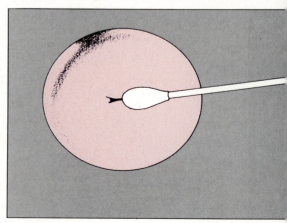

3 When the speculum is fully inserted, open the blades and turn on the illuminator. (For clarity's sake, we've omitted the illuminator in these illustrations.)

As you look through the speculum's opening, you'll see the cervix and part of the vaginal wall (see inset). If you don't see the cervix, move the speculum forward or to either side until you do. *Note:* In some cases, you may have to withdraw the speculum and reinsert it to see the cervix.

4 If everything's OK, the cervix will appear pink and smooth. However, if your patient's pregnant, her cervix will look purplish.

Now, estimate the diameter of your patient's cervix. As you probably know, it should be ¾" to 1¼" (1.9 to 3 cm) in a woman who *has never* given birth by vaginal delivery. If your patient *has* given birth by vaginal delivery, expect the cervix to be about 1¼" to 2" (3 to 5 cm) in diameter.

Observe the cervical os. As shown in the illustrations at left, it should appear circular in a woman who *has never* given birth by vaginal delivery; and stellate in a woman who *has* given birth by vaginal delivery.

Also note the position of the cervix, which may alert you to possible uterine displacement explained on page 119.

5 Now, use the cotton swabs you've collected to obtain specimens for cervical cytology. To do this, moisten a swab with *saline* solution. Then, insert one end of it into the cervical os, and roll the other end several times between your fingers. Withdraw the swab, and wipe it gently against a glass slide. Prepare the slide with Cyto-Prep™ fixative. Label the slide with your patient's name, identification number, and the date. Mark the slide *cervical* sample.

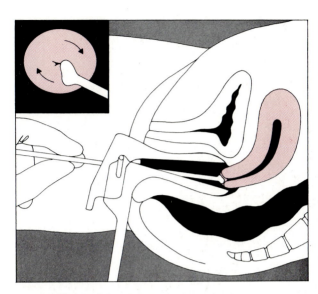

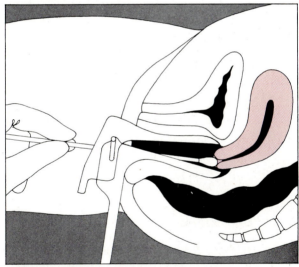

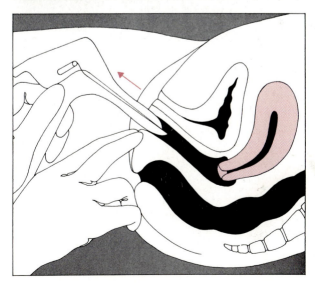

6 Next, use the bifid spatula to scrape cells from the cervix. To do this, insert the spatula into your patient's vagina so the long end of it is on the cervical os.

Position the shorter end of the spatula so it touches the ectocervix.

[Inset] Press down on the spatula, and rotate it 360°. Remove it, and smear the samples on a clean slide. Prepare the slide with fixative, and label.

Using another cotton swab moistened in saline solution, remove some cells from the vaginal wall, just *below* the cervix. Roll the cotton swab between your fingers. Then, withdraw the swab, and prepare a slide, as before. Label the slide with your patient's name, identification number, and the date. Mark the slide *vaginal* sample.

7 Now, insert a cotton swab into the cervical os to obtain cells for a gonorrheal culture. Hold the swab in the cervical os for 10 seconds and withdraw it. Smear the swab on an Agar plate. Label the plate with your patient's name, identification number, and the date. Mark the plate *cervical* sample.

8 You're now ready to remove the vaginal speculum. To do this, slowly close the blades as you pull the speculum toward you.

While you're removing the speculum, inspect the vaginal walls. If all's well, the vaginal mucosa will appear pink and moist. Note any masses, redness, discharge, or ulcerations.

Important: Make sure the speculum's blades are completely closed before you remove it from the vagina.

Document your findings in your nurses' notes.

GU and reproductive systems

Using bimanual palpation to examine your patient's vagina, uterus, and ovaries

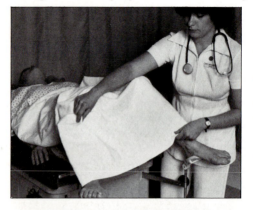

1 *Suppose you're using palpation to examine your patient's vagina, uterus, and ovaries. First, explain the examination procedure to your patient. Make sure she's comfortable and in the lithotomy position.*

The nurse in this photostory will be using her left hand to internally palpate a normally positioned uterus. As you know, a normally positioned uterus tilts forward above the bladder, in front of the rectum. (See the chart on page 119.)

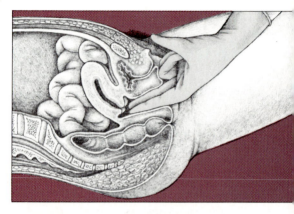

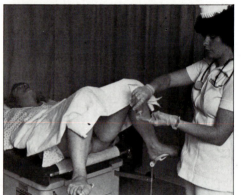

2 Now, slip a pair of gloves on your hands. Using water-soluble jelly, lubricate the index and the middle fingers of your left hand.

Note: If you prefer using your right hand internally, lubricate your right index and middle fingers.

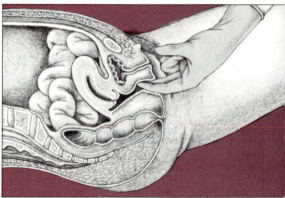

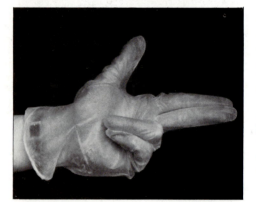

3 Now, position your left hand for vaginal insertion. To do this, curl your left ring and little fingers toward your left palm. Then, put your left index and middle fingers together and abduct your thumb, as shown here. Place your hand at your patient's vaginal opening.

Tell your patient you're getting ready to insert your fingers into her vagina.

🔖 *Nursing tip:* Before you insert your fingers into her vagina, reassure and relax your patient by gently touching her inner thigh.

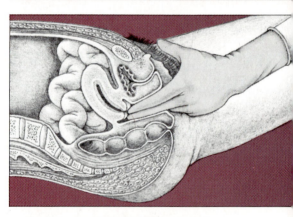

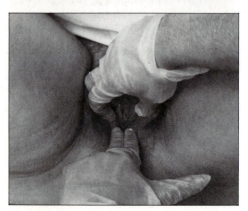

4 Spread apart her labia majora with the thumb and index finger of your right hand. Then, slowly insert the index and middle fingers of your *left* hand into your patient's vagina. Gently press these fingers toward the back of the vaginal canal to avoid irritating the sensitive anterior vaginal wall and urethra.

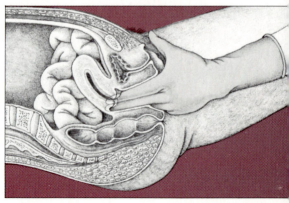

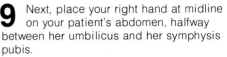

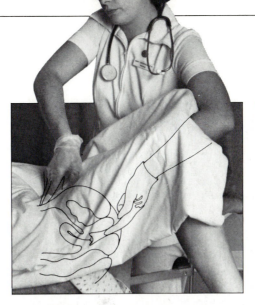

5 When your fingers are fully inserted in your patient's vagina, rotate your hand to a *palm up* position. As you do, palpate the vaginal walls with your fingers. Note any tenderness, nodules, or deviations.

6 Next, sweep your fingers along the anterior vaginal wall, toward the vaginal opening. You should feel the urethra, which is soft and tubular. Palpate the urethra, noting any discharge or tenderness.

Instruct your patient to contract her vaginal muscles around your fingers. If she has good muscle tone, you'll feel her vaginal walls grip your fingers.

7 Now, palpate your patient's cervix. To do this, sweep your fingers from side to side across the cervix and around the os. The cervix should feel moist, smooth, and firm but still be resilient. It should protrude from ½" to 1¼" (1.3 to 3 cm) into her vagina.

8 As you know, the recessed area surrounding the cervix is known as the fornix. Place your fingers in all the fornices and gently move the cervix. If everything's OK, the cervix will move ½" to ¾" (1.3 to 1.9 cm) in any direction. If your patient complains of pain during this part of the procedure, she may have a uterine or an adnexa inflammation.

9 Next, place your right hand at midline on your patient's abdomen, halfway between her umbilicus and her symphysis pubis.

Press downward on your patient's abdomen, toward your left hand. As you do, keep your left hand in a straight line with your forearm. Exert pressure on your patient's perineum with the flexed fingers of your left hand to lift the uterus into a position for palpation.

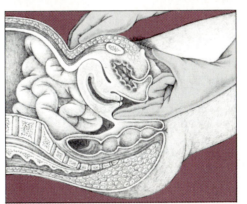

10 Now, slip the fingers of your left hand into your patient's *anterior* fornix. When you do, you should feel part of the posterior uterine wall with your right hand. The fingertips of your left hand should feel part of the anterior uterine wall.

As you palpate the uterus, you should feel a firm, smooth surface under your fingertips. Note any nodules or masses.

11 Next, slip your fingers into your patient's *posterior* fornix. Press upward and forward to bring the anterior uterine wall up to your right hand. Use your left hand to palpate the lower posterior uterine wall. Note any nodules or masses, as before.

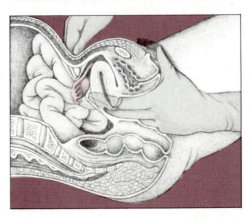

12 Now, move your right hand to your patient's lower right abdominal quadrant. Slip the fingers of your left hand into your patient's right lateral fornix. As you press your right hand toward your left hand, you may feel your patient's right ovary against your left fingertips.

If the ovary is palpable, note its size, shape, and contour. If everything's OK, the ovary will be about 1½" (3.8 cm) long, movable, oval-shaped, firm, and smooth or slightly nodular.

Next, try to locate your patient's left ovary, and palpate it. Note any abnormalities.

Document all your findings in your notes.

GU and reproductive systems

Bimanual rectovaginal palpation

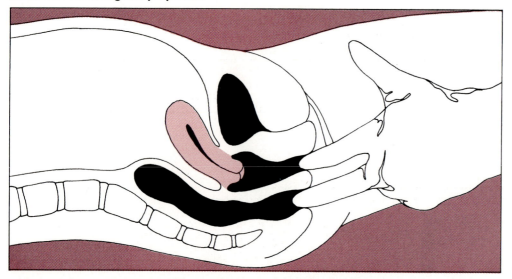

1 *Here's the procedure for performing bimanual rectovaginal palpation.* When you're using this technique, be sure to wear a clean glove on your left hand to prevent possible contamination of your patient's rectum.

Explain the procedure to your patient, and warn her that she may feel some discomfort. Then, lubricate the middle and index fingers of this hand with water-soluble jelly.

Now, instruct your patient to bear down with her vaginal and rectal muscles. As she does, insert your left middle finger into her rectum and your left index finger a little way into her vagina. Use your middle finger to assess your patient's rectal muscles and sphincter tone.

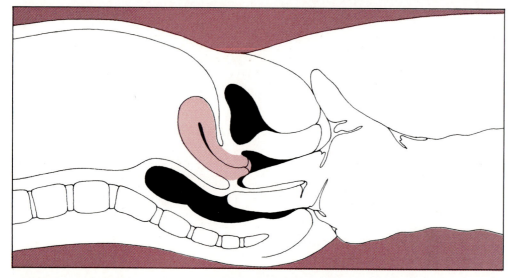

2 Then, insert your fingers deeper. As you do, palpate your patient's rectal wall with your middle finger. It should feel smooth, with resilience in the rectovaginal septum.

When your fingers are fully inserted, gently squeeze the rectovaginal septum between them. It should be free of lumps, masses, deviations, and tenderness.

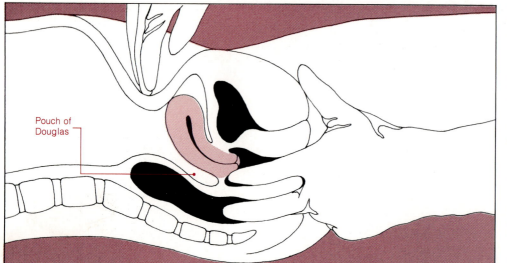

Pouch of Douglas

3 Now, without removing your left hand, place your right hand on your patient's abdomen (at the symphysis pubis) and palpate deeply. Hopefully, you'll feel the posterior edge of your patient's cervix and the lower posterior wall of her uterus against your left index finger. With the middle finger of your left hand, you should be able to palpate the upper posterior wall of your patient's uterus through her rectal wall. Note any lumps, masses, or tenderness.

As you continue to palpate deeply with your right hand, probe deeper with your left fingertips to locate the pouch of Douglas, as shown in this illustration. On palpation, the pouch of Douglas should be nontender.

Finally, document your findings in your nurses' notes.

Identifying uterine displacements

Uterine position	Cervical position	Bimanual palpation findings with fingers placed on abdomen	Bimanual palpation findings with fingers inserted in vagina	Rectovaginal exam findings
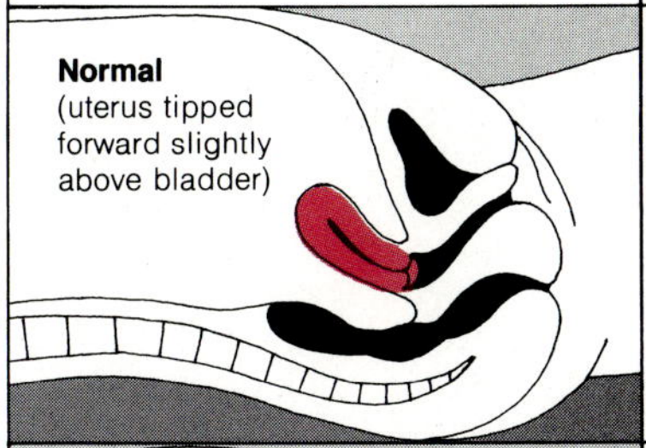 **Normal** (uterus tipped forward slightly above bladder)	• Tipped slightly downward	• Up to ¼ of posterior uterine wall palpable • Up to ½ of anterior uterine wall palpable	• Up to ¾ of anterior uterine wall palpable • Up to ½ of lower posterior uterine wall palpable in posterior fornix	• Pouch of Douglas palpable • Posterior uterine wall palpable
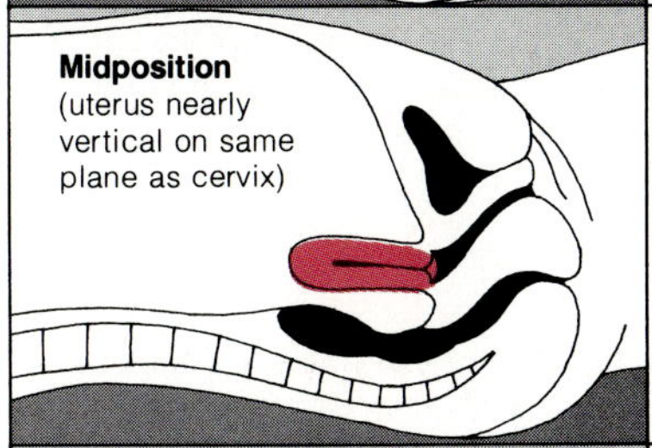 **Midposition** (uterus nearly vertical on same plane as cervix)	• Pointing straight forward	• Fingers in anterior fornix palpable • Uterine wall usually not palpable	• Fingers on abdomen palpable • Lower ¼ of posterior uterine wall palpable in posterior fornix • Lower ¼ of anterior uterine wall palpable with downward pressure in anterior fornix	• Posterior edge of cervix palpable • Pouch of Douglas palpable
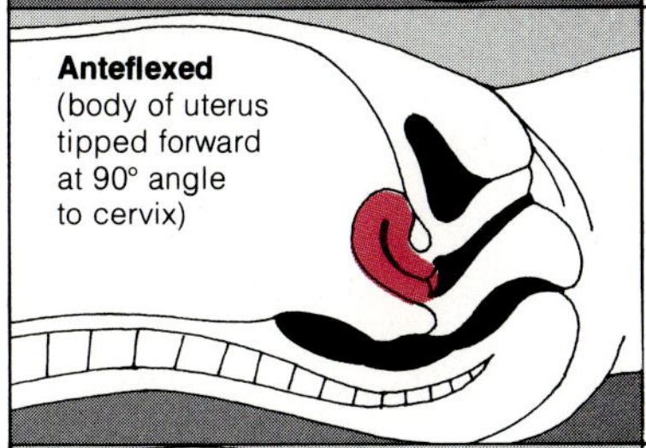 **Anteflexed** (body of uterus tipped forward at 90° angle to cervix)	• Tipped downward	• Upper ½ of posterior uterine wall palpable • In extreme anteflexion, fundus may not be palpable	• Up to ½ of posterior uterine wall palpable • Uterine fundus palpable in anterior fornix • Anterior uterine wall not palpable • With extreme anteflexion, fingers on abdomen palpable	• Small portion of posterior cervix palpable • Pouch of Douglas palpable
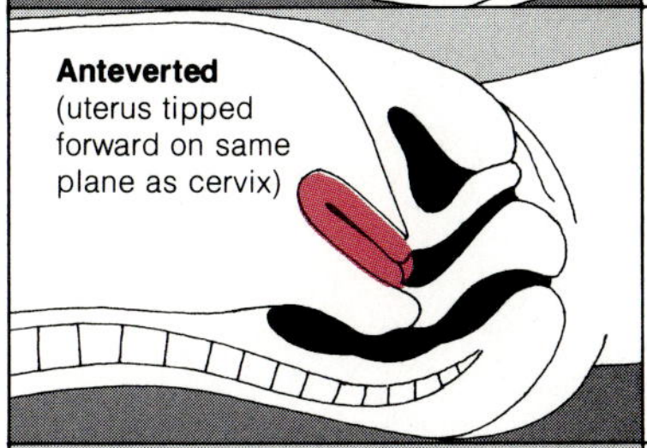 **Anteverted** (uterus tipped forward on same plane as cervix)	• Tipped downward	• Up to ½ of anterior uterine wall palpable • Upper ¼ of posterior fundus palpable	• Up to ¾ of lower anterior uterine wall palpable • Up to ½ of lower posterior uterine wall palpable in posterior fornix	• Posterior edge of cervix palpable • Pouch of Douglas palpable
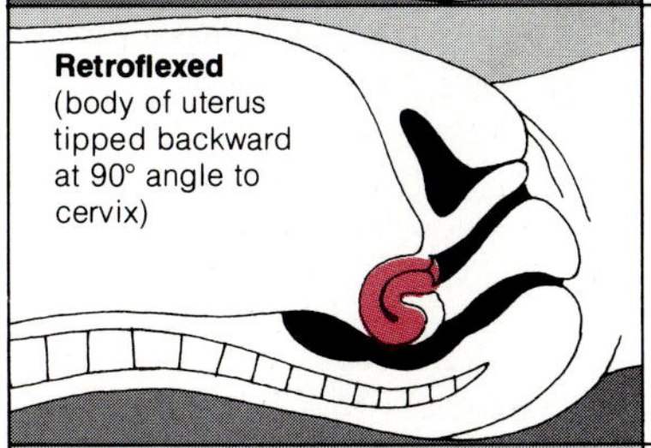 **Retroflexed** (body of uterus tipped backward at 90° angle to cervix)	• Tipped upward	• Fingers in anterior fornix palpable • Lower ¼ of anterior uterine wall palpable	• Lower ¼ of anterior uterine wall palpable • Uterine fundus palpable in posterior fornix	• Up to ½ anterior uterine wall and posterior cervical wall palpable
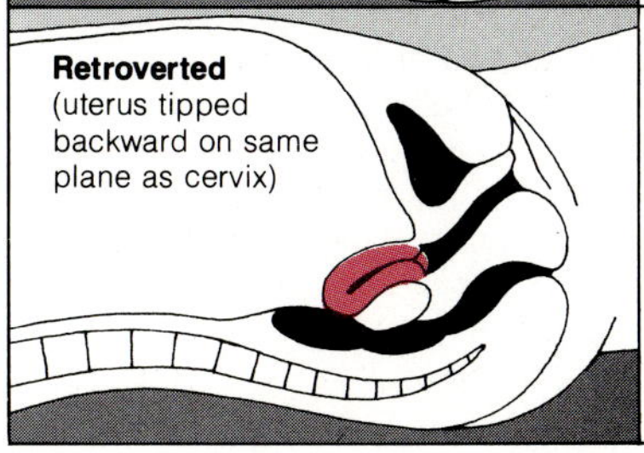 **Retroverted** (uterus tipped backward on same plane as cervix)	• Tipped upward	• Fingers in anterior fornix palpable • Uterine wall not palpable	• Anterior and lower portion of anterior uterine wall palpable • Lower ½ of posterior uterine wall palpable in posterior fornix	• Portion of posterior cervix palpable • Pouch of Douglas palpable • Lower ¼ of anterior uterine wall palpable • Lower ¼ of posterior uterine wall palpable

GU and reproductive systems

How to examine your patient's pelvis and groin

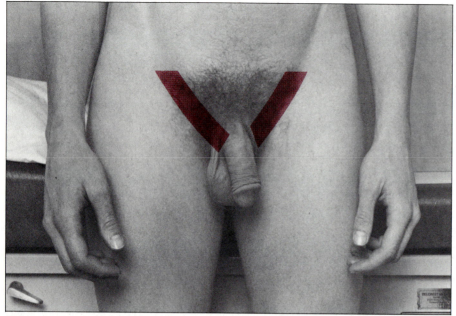

1 *If you're inspecting your patient's pelvis and groin, follow these steps:*
Ask your patient to stand facing you. Position yourself in front of him. (If he's unable to stand, have him lie flat on his back on an exam table.)
Now, observe your patient's pelvis. It should be symmetrical and shaped like an inverted triangle. Note any skin discolorations, lumps, or masses in the pelvic area.
Carefully inspect the groin area indicated by the shaded sections in this photo. As you know, these are the areas where hernias may occur.

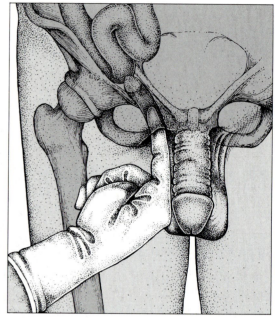

4 Now, move your finger about ½" (1.3 cm) above (and lateral to) the edge of the pubic bone. You'll feel the triangular-shaped opening of the external inguinal ring.
If all's well, the inguinal ring will be unobstructed. If you feel a mass protruding through your patient's inguinal opening, suspect an inguinal hernia.

2 Next, palpate your patient's right inguinal area. Note any lumps or bulges. Then, ask your patient to bear down as you continue to palpate. Feel for lumps, bulges, or a sliding sensation against your fingertips.
Then, examine your patient's right inguinal ring, as the nurse is doing here. To do this, place your right index finger on your patient's scrotum, slightly below his penis, to the right.

3 Now, gently push upward at a 45° angle, to infold the loose skin of your patient's scrotum. *Important:* Never pinch the skin of the scrotum, or the spermatic cord. Doing so will cause your patient extreme pain.
Carefully insert your finger into the patient's inguinal ring, along the spermatic cord's path. When your finger's fully inserted, you should feel the pubic bone with your fingertip.

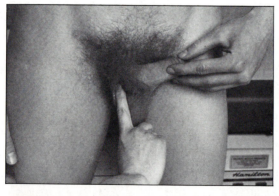

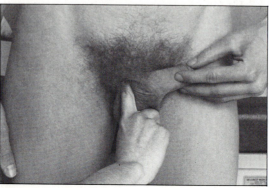

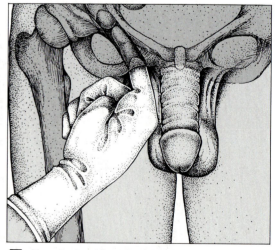

5 Now, instruct your patient to bear down and cough. When he does, you may feel a sliding sensation of tissue against your fingertip. This indicates a hernia *above* your patient's inguinal ring, as shown in this illustration.
If tissue strikes the *side* of your finger, your patient probably has a direct hernia. If tissue strikes the *tip* of your finger, he may have an indirect hernia.
Document your findings in your nurses' notes.

Inspecting and palpating your patient's penis

1 *Examining your patient's penis? First, slip a pair of gloves on your hands, as the nurse is doing here. Then, ask your patient to stand facing you.*

[Inset] If your patient can't stand up, instruct him to lie flat on his back on an exam table. Then, stand at his side for the exam.

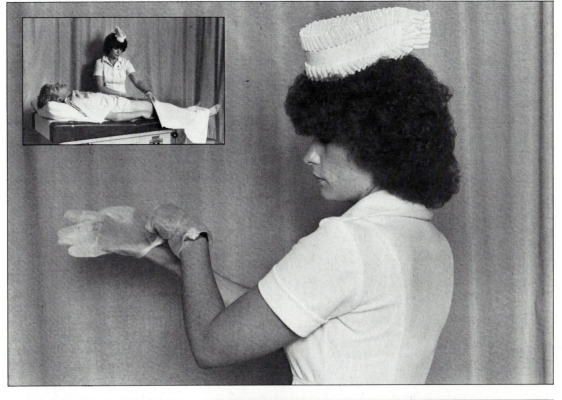

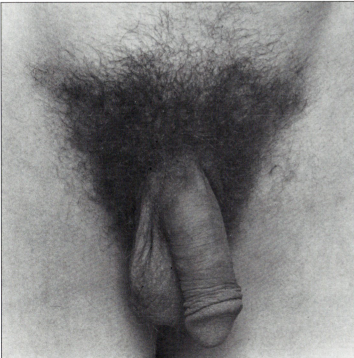

2 Observe your patient's pubic hair. It should be thickest at his symphysis pubis and extend over his inner thighs and scrotum. In some patients, a line of hair may extend upward, toward the umbilicus. Note any bald or sparse patches in the pubic area.

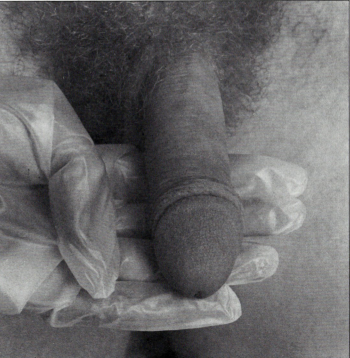

3 Next, observe your patient's penis. Is your patient circumcised? If so, his glans penis will be exposed, and you'll see a ridge of tissue at its base. If he's uncircumcised, his glans will be covered by foreskin.

GU and reproductive systems

Inspecting and palpating your patient's penis continued

4 Observe the anterior surface of your patient's penis. Then, lift his penis up to check its posterior surface. If everything's OK, the entire penis will look pink and smooth. Note any ulcers, swelling, scars, nodules, or skin discolorations.

Palpate any abnormalities with your index and middle fingers.

As you know, the urethral orifice should be located at the *tip* of your patient's penis. If it's located elsewhere, document this abnormality in your nurses' notes.

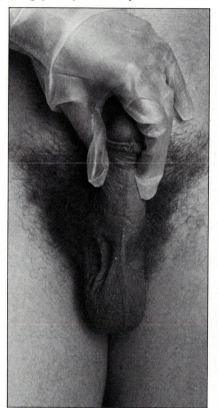

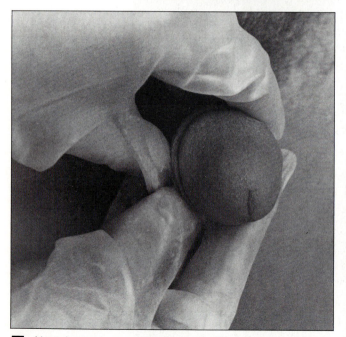

5 Next, inspect your patient's glans. If he's uncircumcised, you'll need to retract his foreskin, as described on the page opposite.

The glans should look pink, smooth, and cone-shaped. Note any lesions, hardness, growths, swelling, or inflammation.

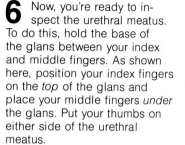

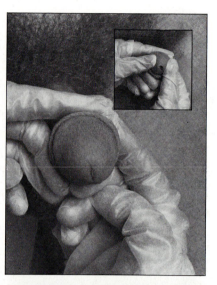

6 Now, you're ready to inspect the urethral meatus. To do this, hold the base of the glans between your index and middle fingers. As shown here, position your index fingers on the *top* of the glans and place your middle fingers *under* the glans. Put your thumbs on either side of the urethral meatus.

[Inset] Then, move your thumbs outward to open the urethral meatus. Inspect the meatus, noting any lesions, strictures, or discharge. If you see a discharge, take a specimen of it for a culture, as described on the page opposite.

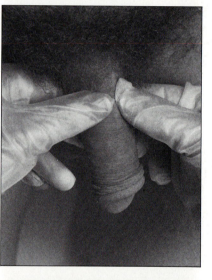

7 Next, place both thumbs and index fingers at the base of your patient's penis. Position your fingers around the penis to cover as much of its surface as you can.

8 Now, slide your fingers down your patient's penis, to the base of the glans.

As you do, rotate your fingers slightly from side to side, to palpate the entire penis. If all's well, the penis will feel soft but not flabby (unless your patient's elderly). Note any thickening, nodules, protrusions, or hardness.

Suppose, following palpation, you notice a discharge from the urethral meatus. Take a specimen of it for a culture.

Finally, document all your findings in your nurses' notes.

How to retract a penile foreskin

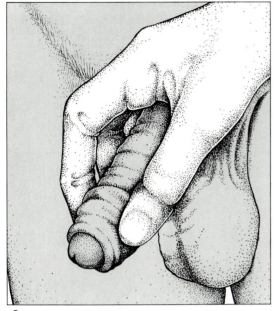

1 *If your patient's uncircumcised, you'll need to retract his foreskin to visualize his glans.*
To do this, place your thumb and index finger on either side of your patient's glans, as shown.

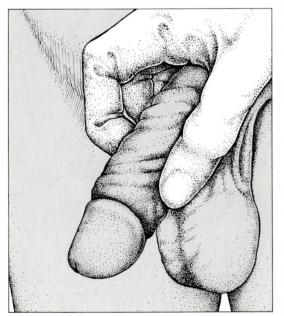

2 Using gentle pressure, draw the foreskin back over the penile shaft. Your patient's foreskin should slide back easily. If it doesn't, your patient may have phimosis (constriction of the foreskin over the glans).

Suppose your patient's foreskin doesn't cover his glans but is constricted behind it. He may have paraphimosis (retracted foreskin).

Immediately notify the doctor of any abnormality. Document your findings in your nurses' notes.

How to culture a penile discharge

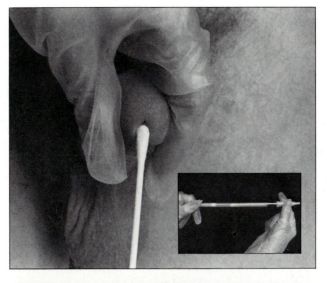

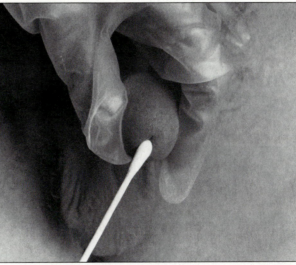

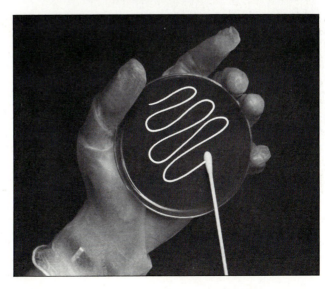

1 *What if you notice a discharge from your patient's penis? Document its color, consistency, and odor. Then, to check for bacterial growth, take two separate specimens for cultures, as explained here.*

To do this, first roll a sterile cotton swab in the discharge. Then, place the swab in a Culturette™ tube, as the nurse has done in the inset photo.

2 With a second sterile cotton swab, get another specimen for a gonorrheal culture.

3 Then, brush this swab over an Agar plate's surface, as the nurse is doing here. Finally, label both cultures, and send them to the lab for analyses.

GU and reproductive systems

Inspecting and palpating your patient's scrotum

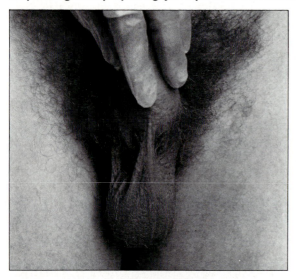

1 *To inspect your patient's scrotum, have him stand facing you, as you position yourself in front of him. Then, gently support his penis against his symphysis pubis, to visualize his scrotum.*

Observe your patient's scrotum carefully. His scrotal sac should look almost symmetrical except for the left side, which usually hangs slightly lower. The scrotal skin should appear wrinkled and firmly hug the testicles.

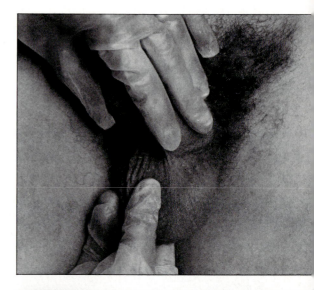

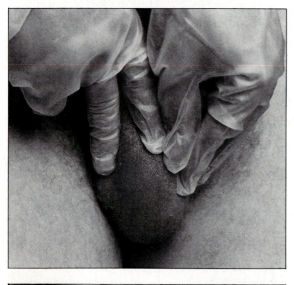

2 Now, observe both the anterior and posterior surfaces of the scrotum. Note any swelling, nodules, inflammation, ulcers, or distended veins.

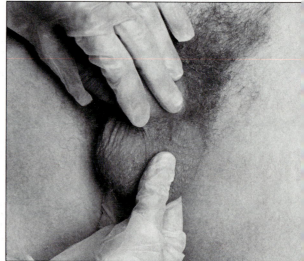

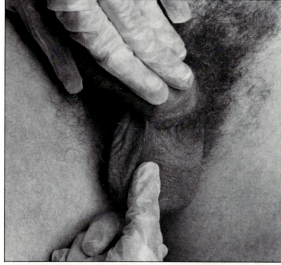

3 Next, prepare to palpate your patient's scrotum. To do this, place your right index finger on the scrotum's right posterior surface. Place your right thumb on the right anterior surface.

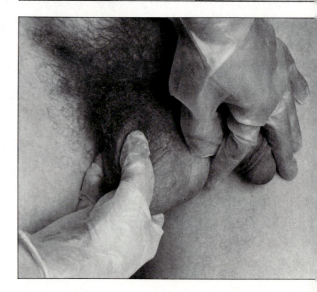

4 Press your fingers together to palpate for your patient's right testicle. Remember to palpate *gently*, since squeezing will cause your patient extreme pain.

If the testicle's present, it should feel smooth, firm, rubbery, and slightly tender, and should be movable within the scrotal sac. A patient over age 50 may have testicles that feel shrunken and soft.

5 Suppose the testicle is not there or isn't fully descended into the scrotal sac. Note this carefully, and document it in your nurses' notes.

Palpate for your patient's left testicle in the same manner, as shown here. Both testicles should be similar in size, shape, and consistency.

Did you discover an abnormal mass in your patient's scrotum? If so, try to press your fingers together *above* the mass. Do your fingers meet? The mass is probably contained in the scrotum. If your fingers *don't* meet, the mass may extend downward from his abdomen, indicating an indirect hernia. Document your findings, and notify the doctor.

6 Now, palpate both of your patient's spermatic cords. To locate the cord, gently grasp your patient's right testicle between your right thumb and index finger. Then, slide your fingers up to the testicle's top.

Extending from the top of the testicle, you'll feel a smooth, round, cordlike structure that's firm but resilient. This is the spermatic cord. If you feel a soft, movable, mass along the cord, suspect an accumulation of fluid (hydrocele of the cord). A grouping of hard, nodular, cordlike structures along the cord indicates varioceles, varices, or varicose veins.

Document your findings.

How to transilluminate your patient's scrotum

1 *Have you detected a lump or mass in your patient's scrotum? If so, use transillumination to evaluate it.*

Begin by placing a lamp beside you, so you can see after the room's darkened. Turn on the lamp; then darken the rest of the room.

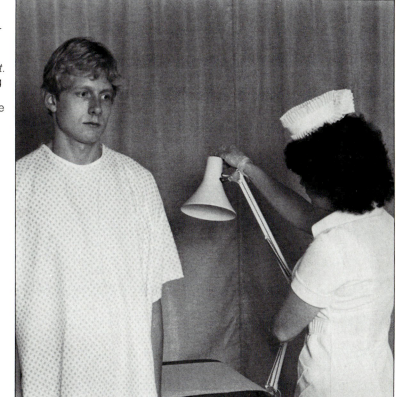

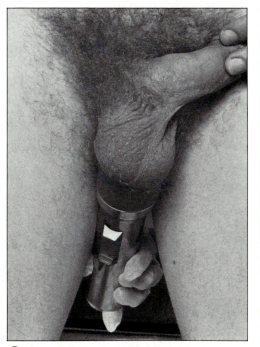

2 Now, place a flashlight behind what you suspect is the affected side of the scrotum. Try to place the flashlight head as flat as possible against the scrotum's posterior surface.

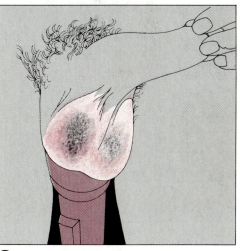

3 Next, turn off the lamp beside you, and switch on your flashlight. Observe the scrotum's anterior surface.

If everything's OK, the scrotum will transilluminate with a red glow. The testicle will appear as an opaque oval shadow. Lumps, masses, or blood-filled areas will also look like opaque shadows.

Transilluminate the opposite side of your patient's scrotum, and compare the results.

Then, document your findings, specifically, in your nurses' notes.

GU and reproductive systems

Using palpation to examine your patient's rectum, prostate gland, and seminal vesicles

1 *Do you know how to examine your patient's rectum, prostate gland, and seminal vesicles? If you're unsure, study the guidelines in this photostory.*

First, instruct your patient to urinate. Then, slip gloves on your hands. Lubricate the index finger you'll use to examine your patient's rectum with water-soluble jelly.

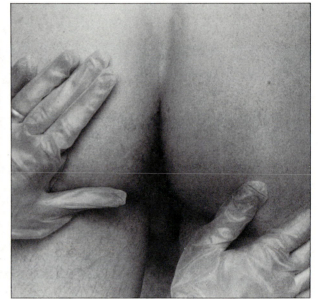

2 Next, ask your patient to stand facing the end of an exam table. Instruct him to bend over and rest his upper torso on the table.

[Inset] Suppose your patient can't stand. Have him lie on his left side, with his back facing you. Position his buttocks at the edge of the exam table. Then, instruct him to draw up his knees toward his chest.

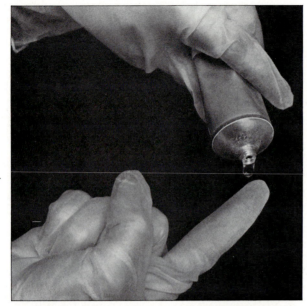

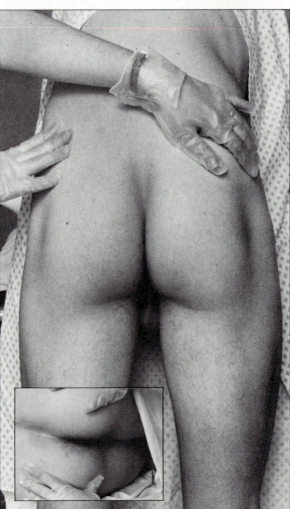

3 Now, spread apart your patient's buttocks by gently pushing his left buttock outward with your left hand.

Examine the area between his buttocks for lumps, inflammation, or skin tears. Your patient's anal opening should appear puckered and brown.

Then, tell your patient to bear down, as if he were moving his bowels. As he does, observe the anal opening for protrusions. Reddish protrusions made up of distended veins indicate hemorrhoids. However, if you see reddish, velvety-looking tissue projecting from his anus, suspect prolapsed rectal mucosa. Describe any anal protrusions in your nurses' notes.

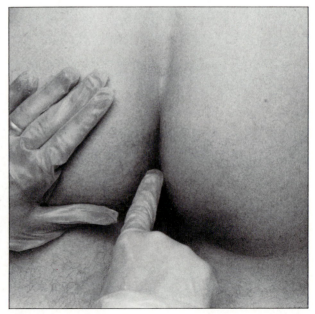

4 Next, place your gloved index finger at the base of your patient's anal opening. Instruct him to bear down, to reduce sphincter tension.

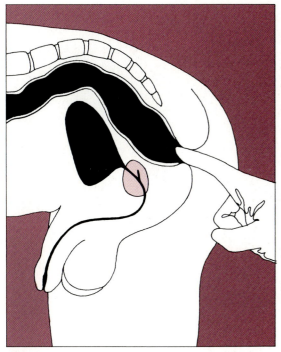

5 Now, gently slide the first joint of your lubricated finger into your patient's anus. Note the tone of your patient's sphincter muscle. Expect it to feel tight, not flabby.

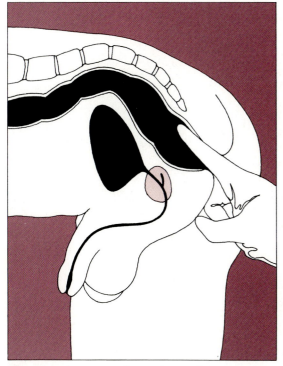

6 Then, insert your finger deeper into your patient's rectum. As you do, palpate the anterior rectal wall by moving your finger from side to side.

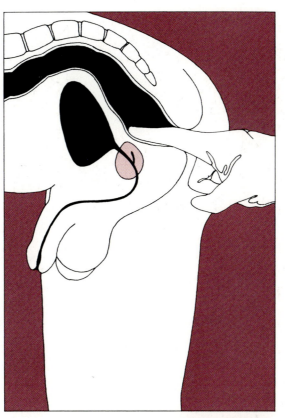

7 If your patient's prostate gland is still intact, you'll feel it through the anterior rectal wall, located about 2" (5 cm) from the rectal opening. If all's well, it should be a smooth, rubbery-feeling, nontender mass.

Does your patient's prostate gland protrude more than ½" (1.3 cm) into his rectum? If so, document the amount of protrusion as: Grade 1, ½" to ¾" (1.3 to 1.9 cm); Grade 2, ¾" to 1¼" (1.9 to 3.1 cm); Grade 3, 1¼" to 1¾" (3.1 to 4.4 cm); or Grade 4, 1¾" (4.4 cm) or more.

Now, estimate the prostate gland's size. It should be about 1¾" (4.4 cm) in diameter.

Document the appropriate grade of prostate gland protrusion, as well as the gland's size, shape, and consistency.

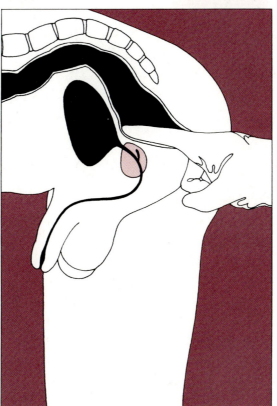

8 Next, place your finger on the anterior rectal wall, slightly above the prostate gland. Palpate for your patient's seminal vesicles, but don't expect to feel them unless they're inflamed.

Continue to palpate the anterior rectal wall, as before. Palpate as much of it as your finger can reach. Then, rotate your hand, palm up. Palpate the posterior rectal wall as you slide your finger down toward the anal opening. Note any lumps, ulcerations, or tenderness.

GU and reproductive systems

Using palpation to examine your patient's rectum, prostate gland, and seminal vesicles continued

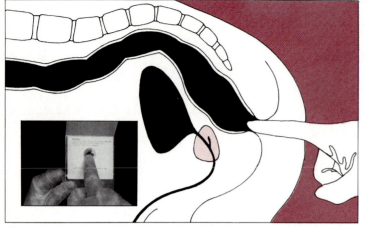

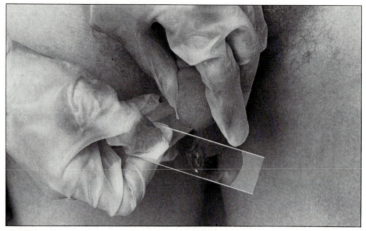

9 When you reach the anal opening, withdraw your finger completely. Inspect it for traces of blood, which indicate rectal bleeding.

[Inset] What if you have feces on your finger? Smear the feces on a Hemocult® slide. Then, label the slide properly, and send it to the lab, to check for occult bleeding.

Now, cleanse your patient's rectum with a cleansing tissue, to remove traces of feces and lubricant. Remove your glove, and dispose of it.

10 Finally, check your patient's urethral meatus for any discharge that may be caused by prostate palpation. To do this, put on a pair of clean gloves and ask your patient to stand facing you. Then, follow the guidelines on page 122 to open his urethral meatus.

Suppose you see a discharge. Place a glass slide under his meatus to collect a drop. Send the properly labeled slide to the lab for microscopic examination.

Document the procedure, including your findings, in your notes.

Identifying GU problems

DANGER SIGNS

Assessment variables	Nonpenetrating renal injury	Renal colic	Acute pyelo-nephritis	Acute bacterial cystitis	Urethral stricture
Pain	• Upper abdominal or flank tenderness	• Severe flank pain radiating across abdomen to groin	• Pain in one or both flanks • Dysuria	• Dysuria • Possible suprapubic discomfort and low back pain	• None (unless urethritis, cystitis, or hydronephrosis is present)
Urination difficulties	• Possible hematuria	• Possible hematuria • Frequency	• Dysuria • Frequent, urgent need to urinate • Urine may be bloody, cloudy, and foul-smelling	• Dysuria • Frequent, urgent need to urinate • Nocturia • Possible hematuria	• Difficulty starting urination • Force and size of urine stream decreased • Frequent, urgent need to urinate if infection is present
Palpation	• Mass may be felt in flank.	• Possible extreme tenderness over posterior flank • Tenderness over the affected ureter	• Tenderness of costovertebral angle over affected kidney • Affected kidney may be enlarged.	• Suprapubic tenderness	• Lumps may be felt on urethral membrane. • Mass in suprapubic area may indicate distended bladder from urinary retention.
Special	• Possible external flank contusion	• Possible nausea, vomiting, diaphoresis, and pallor • Possible chills and fever	• May be asymptomatic • Chills, fever, and weakness • Some abdominal rigidity	• Patient is usually afebrile.	• Possible infection from urinary retention

Identifying female reproductive disorders

Assessment variables	Cancer of the cervix	Uterine fibroid	Gonorrhea
Pain	• Pain is late symptom.	• Dysmenorrhea, backache, or possible discomfort in lower abdomen.	• Usually none, although sometimes patient has mild abdominal discomfort.
Discharge	• Whitish uterine discharge becomes dark and foul-smelling as condition worsens • Irregular vaginal bleeding between periods or after menopause	• Irregular vaginal bleeding between periods or after menopause	• Slight purulent vaginal discharge possible
Palpation	• Nontender abdomen • In early stage, mass not palpable.	• Mass may be felt above symphysis pubis.	• Bartholin's glands may be swollen and tender.
Special	• Granular ulceration at or near the cervical os becomes larger, as condition worsens • In late stage, signs of metastasis; for example, weight loss, weakness, anemia, back and leg pain	• Condition may be asymptomatic. • Possible constipation and urinary retention	• If bladder is involved, need to urinate is frequent and urgent. • May lead to pelvic inflammatory disease (PID), with fever, abdominal pain, nausea, and vomiting

Identifying male reproductive disorders

Assessment variables	Acute pyogenic orchitis	Cancer of the prostate	Gonorrhea
Pain	• Sudden, severe pain in affected testicle, radiating to inguinal canal	• Pain is late symptom.	• Burning urination • Possible extreme pain in urethral meatus
Discharge	• None	• Usually none	• Urethral discharge is profuse and mucopurulent.
Palpation	• Affected testicle is swollen, tense, and tender.	• Hard, irregular nodule on prostate (usually on posterior lobe). In early stage, nodule is mobile, becoming harder and fixed as condition worsens.	• Urethral tenderness • In some cases, lymph glands are tender and enlarged.
Special	• Scrotum may be red and swollen. • Possible high fever, nausea, and vomiting	• Urinary obstruction may cause hesitancy. • Size and force of urine stream decreased • Frequent urge to void • Nocturia • In late stage, signs of metastasis; for example, weight loss, anemia, oliguria, and lumbosacral pain	• Penis may be red and swollen. • As infection spreads, need to urinate is frequent and urgent. • Urine may be bloody and contain pus.

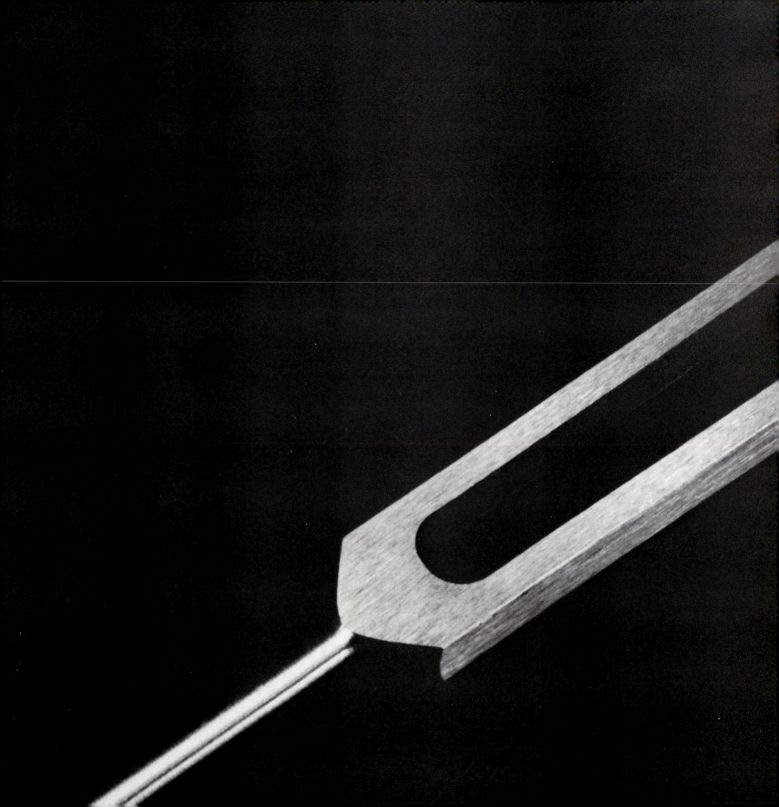

Evaluating the Brain and Spinal Cord

Nervous system

Nervous system

DOCUMENTING

When you perform a neurologic assessment on your patient, you'll want to know how to test your patient's cerebellar function, muscle tone, and muscle strength.

Do you know how to perform the Romberg test? Or test your patient's tactile discrimination? Do you know how to locate and test her Achilles tendon reflex?

In the next few pages, we'll answer these questions and show you how to do each of these tests. Chances are, you won't perform all of these tests on your patient. However, we've included them all as a handy reference.

Be sure to read the material carefully.

Neurologic questions: What to ask

Before you can properly assess your patient's nervous system, you must obtain pertinent baseline data. To do this, interview your patient carefully, using the questions below as a guideline:

• Do you suffer from frequent headaches? If so, do they seem to follow a pattern? Describe the details. What medication (if any) do you take to relieve them? Have you been treated by a doctor for your headaches?
• How would you rate your muscle strength? Good? Average? Below average? Or poor? Why?
• Have you noticed any change in muscle strength? If so, when did you first notice it?
• Do you have paralysis or weakness in any part of your body? If so, where? When did you first notice it? Describe the details.
• Do you ever have tremors, spasms, or shakiness in your muscles? If so, how often do they occur? Have you been treated by a doctor for this condition?
• Do you have problems with your balance? Have you ever fallen because you've lost your balance?
• How would you rate your muscle coordination? Excellent? Good? Fair? Or poor? Why?
• Do you ever have seizures? If so, how often? Does anything seem to bring them on? Do you take any medication for the condition? If so, what do you take, and how often do you take it?
• Has your doctor told you that you have epilepsy? If so, when? Describe the details. What medication (if any) do you take?
• Do you drop things frequently? If so, are you doing it more often recently? Describe the details.

• Do you ever burn or cut yourself without realizing it? Describe the details.
• Have you noticed any change in your ability to feel textures? If so, describe the details.
• Have you noticed a change in your ability to concentrate? Do you get bored easily? Do you have difficulty following conversations or television shows?
• How good is your memory? Have you noticed a change in your ability to remember things? If so, describe the details.
• Do you ever faint or black out (even for a few moments)? If so, how often? Are there ever blocks of time that you can't recall?
• Do you ever have difficulty speaking or expressing the words you're thinking? For example, do you know what you want to say but can't seem to get it out?
• Have you ever had a stroke? If so, describe the details.
• Have you ever been treated by a neurologist or a neurosurgeon? If so, explain why. Is the doctor still treating you?
• Have you noticed any changes in your mental awareness, muscle coordination, or sensations?

As you ask your patient these questions, observe her carefully. Look for signs of possible neurologic deficiencies; for example, muscle weakness, ptosis, and confusion. Listen closely to her answers. Does she seem to comprehend what you're asking?

Important: You'll find other pertinent questions to consider in Sections 1 and 2. Review them before you complete this part of your assessment.

Neurologic system: Brain basics

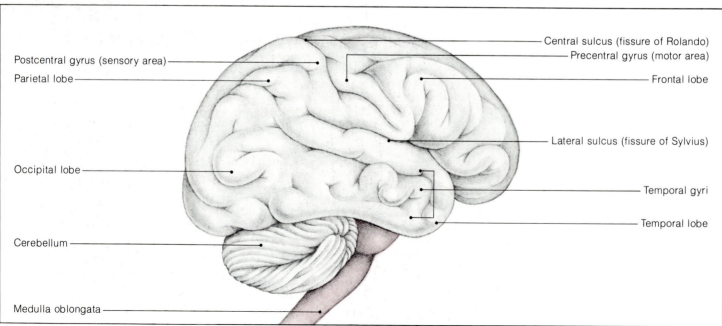

Central sulcus (fissure of Rolando)
Precentral gyrus (motor area)
Postcentral gyrus (sensory area)
Parietal lobe
Frontal lobe
Lateral sulcus (fissure of Sylvius)
Occipital lobe
Temporal gyri
Temporal lobe
Cerebellum
Medulla oblongata

Neurologic system: Spinal cord basics

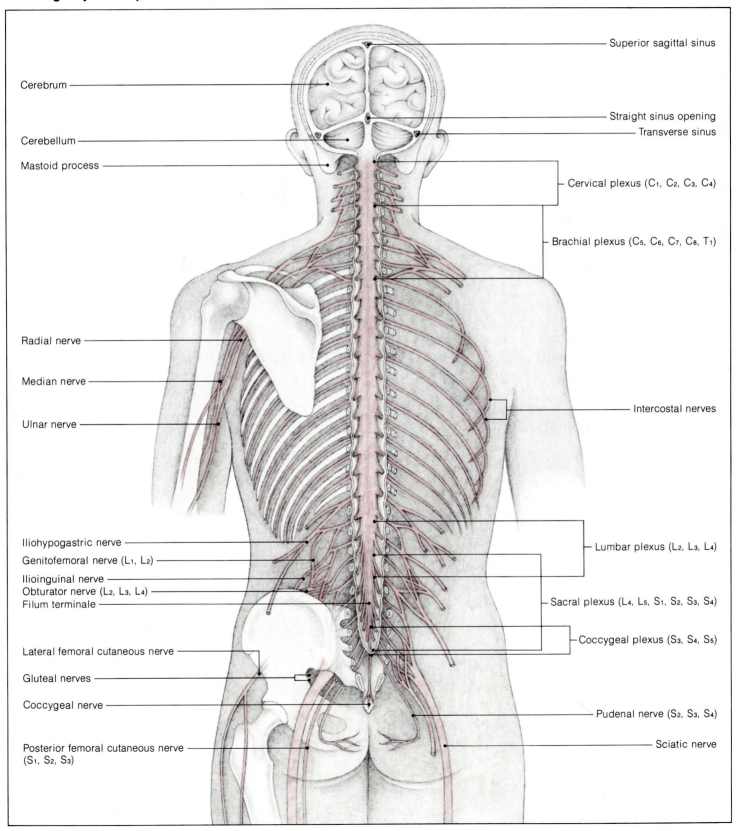

Cerebrum

Cerebellum

Mastoid process

Radial nerve

Median nerve

Ulnar nerve

Iliohypogastric nerve

Genitofemoral nerve (L₁, L₂)

Ilioinguinal nerve

Obturator nerve (L₂, L₃, L₄)

Filum terminale

Lateral femoral cutaneous nerve

Gluteal nerves

Coccygeal nerve

Posterior femoral cutaneous nerve
(S₁, S₂, S₃)

Superior sagittal sinus

Straight sinus opening

Transverse sinus

Cervical plexus (C₁, C₂, C₃, C₄)

Brachial plexus (C₅, C₆, C₇, C₈, T₁)

Intercostal nerves

Lumbar plexus (L₂, L₃, L₄)

Sacral plexus (L₄, L₅, S₁, S₂, S₃, S₄)

Coccygeal plexus (S₃, S₄, S₅)

Pudenal nerve (S₂, S₃, S₄)

Sciatic nerve

Nervous system

How to quickly evaluate your patient's emotional and mental status

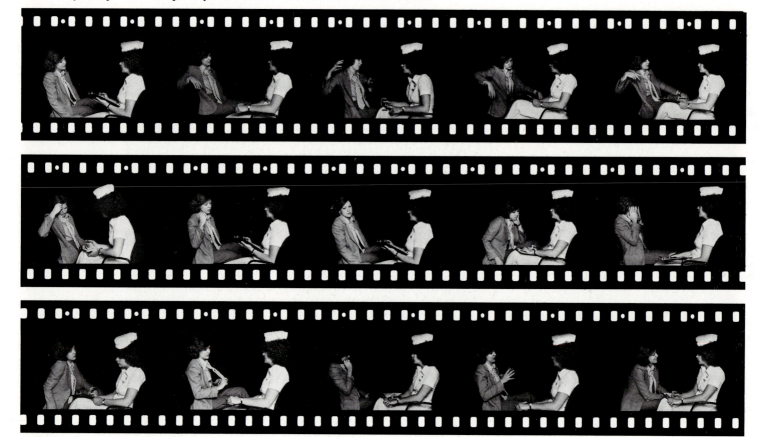

Your patient's behavior and appearance provides you with clues about her emotional and mental status. From the moment you meet, you begin to assess her. Learn how by studying these guidelines. But remember, the end result of your assessment is only one way of evaluating your patient's emotional and mental status. By performing the other tests in this section, you'll gain a more complete view of her neurologic status. If you're unsure of your findings, verify them with another health professional.

As you interview your patient, note how she's dressed. Are her clothes clean, and is the style appropriate for someone her age? Observe her hair, fingernails, and skin. Do they appear clean and cared for?

As your patient speaks, watch her facial expression. Is it appropriate? Then ask yourself how you'd describe it: confused, sad, afraid? If your patient's face has a blank look, her lack of expression may be caused by one or more of the following: preoccupation, mental illness, drug abuse, subnormal intelligence, or facial paralysis.

Note your patient's gestures and other body movements. Are they coordinated and smooth, or jerky?

Does your patient appear alert and interested in what you're saying? Or does she seem dazed, drowsy, and inattentive? Is she able to understand your questions and answer them logically? Or are her answers confused or incoherent?

Encourage your patient to talk about herself. Does she seem satisfied with her life, or pessimistic and depressed (for no reason)? Is her mood even, or does it fluctuate?

Note any preoccupation on her part with certain subjects. Does

she have a complaint she repeats excessively? Does she make inappropriate statements? Is she in touch with reality, or does she see and hear things that aren't there?

Check your patient's distant memory by asking her to tell you her birthdate and the birthdates of loved ones.

To test her recent memory, pick three numbers, and recite them several times. Then ask your patient to repeat them back to you. If she can do this, recite three more numbers, and ask her to repeat these *backward*. Continue this pattern, adding a number each time your patient successfully repeats a series. If all's well, your patient should be able to repeat a series of five to eight numbers forward and four to six backward.

To estimate your patient's general intelligence, perform a quick test of her knowledge and vocabulary. Here's how:

Ask your patient four or five easy questions; for example, *How many objects make up a dozen? Name the four seasons.* If your patient can answer these correctly, ask several complex questions; for example, *Why does oil float on water? What is a hieroglyph?*

Ask your patient to define some words you've selected or to use them in a sentence. Begin with simple words such as ball, penny, novel. If your patient does well with these, continue the test with more difficult words; for example, statutory, reminiscent, relevance.

Now, ask your patient four or five questions to test her judgmental ability. Make up your own questions or use these: *What would you do if you lost something you borrowed from a friend? What would you do if you found a lost child?* Note your patient's ability to solve the problems and to distinguish between right and wrong.

Finally, document the results of these tests in your nurses' notes.

How to test superficial reflexes

1 *To test your patient's superficial reflexes, get a key or applicator stick to gently scratch her skin. Then proceed as follows:*

Make sure your patient's lying on her back on an exam table, with her legs slightly flexed at her knees. Instruct her to place her arms at her sides, and explain the examination procedure.

Now, ask your patient to exhale. As she does, gently draw the key or applicator stick across her upper right abdominal quadrant, from her side toward her umbilicus. Expect her umbilicus to move toward her upper right quadrant. Be sure to note any variations.

Repeat the test on her other three abdominal quadrants.

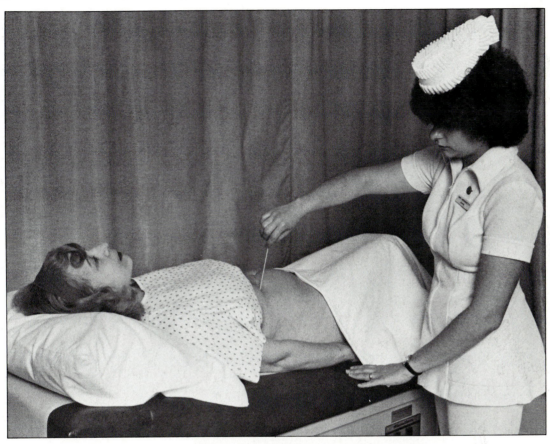

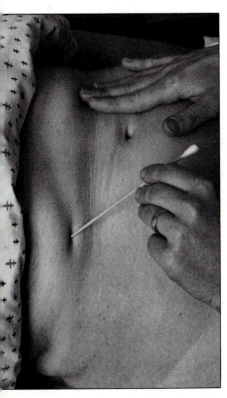

2 Suppose your patient is obese. You may not be able to see her umbilicus move. If so, begin the test by gently drawing her skin and underlying fatty tissue away from the upper right quadrant.

Then, following the same procedure as above, draw the key or applicator stick over her upper right quadrant, noting umbilical movement. Repeat the procedure on the other abdominal quadrants.

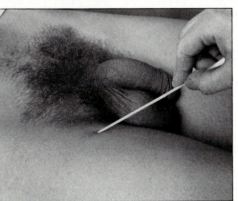

3 If your patient's a man, test his cremasteric reflex. Gently draw the stick down his right groin, then along his right inner thigh. Expect the right cremasteric muscle to contract and the right testicle to rise slightly. Note abnormalities.

Repeat the test on his left side.

4 Finally, test your patient's plantar reflex. Lightly scratch the outer aspect of your patient's right foot from the heel up, as shown here. Her toes should curl *downward*. If they don't, note it carefully.

Then repeat the test on her left foot.

Note: If your patient's big toe dorsiflexes and her other toes fan out, document this as an abnormal Babinski response. The response suggests an organic lesion of the pyramidal tract.

Document all findings from these tests in your nurses' notes.

Nervous system

How to test deep tendon reflexes

1 *Knowing how to test your patient's deep tendon reflexes should be part of your assessment skills. Do you know how? If you're unsure, follow these steps:*

First, instruct your patient to sit on the edge of an exam table. Encourage her to *relax completely.* Then, tell her to hold her right arm about 6" (15.2 cm) away from her side.

Place your left hand on your patient's *right* shoulder. Make sure your thumb is directly over her shoulder tendon.

With your right hand, grasp a reflex hammer and strike your left thumb. If all's well, your patient's right arm will move toward her body. Note any lack of movement.

Repeat the test on your patient's left shoulder.

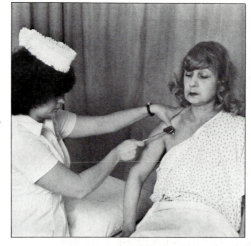

2 To test your patient's bicep reflex, slightly flex her right elbow, as shown here.

Hold your patient's elbow, with your thumb pressing tightly against the bicep muscle tendon. With your right hand, grasp the reflex hammer and strike your thumb. If everything's OK, your patient's bicep muscle will contract, flexing her arm at the elbow.

Repeat the test on your patient's left arm.

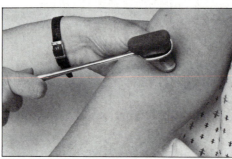

3 Next, test your patient's tricep reflex. To do this, flex your patient's right arm at her elbow and hold her arm at the wrist.

Grasp the reflex hammer with your other hand, and strike the tendon of the tricep muscle directly over the elbow. Expect the tricep muscle to contract, extending your patient's arm at her elbow.

Repeat the test on her left elbow.

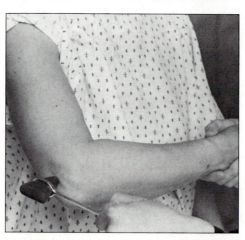

4 Next, hold your patient's right hand slightly below her wrist, and position her palm down. With the reflex hammer, strike the tendon of her brachioradial muscle, which (in most cases) is located about 1" to 2" (2.5 to 5 cm) above the wrist. Her forearm should rotate laterally, so her palm turns upward.

Repeat the test on her left brachioradial muscle.

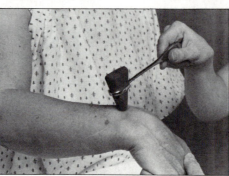

5 Now, test your patient's patellar reflex. Position your right hand slightly above your patient's right knee. With your left hand, grasp the reflex hammer and strike your patient's patellar tendon, just below the patella. Her leg should respond to your action by kicking forward.

Repeat the test on her left knee.

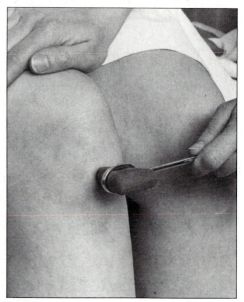

6 To test your patient's Achilles tendon reflex, hold her right foot with your left hand. Gently rotate her foot outward. Strike the Achilles tendon with the reflex hammer. As you do, watch the tricep surae muscle contract (plantar flexion). Then, note how quickly it relaxes after contraction. If all's well, the muscle should relax in about 1 or 2 seconds.

Repeat the test on her left Achilles tendon.

Finally, document the findings from these tests in your nurses' notes.

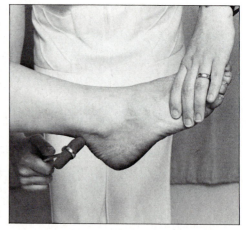

Testing your patient's sensory system

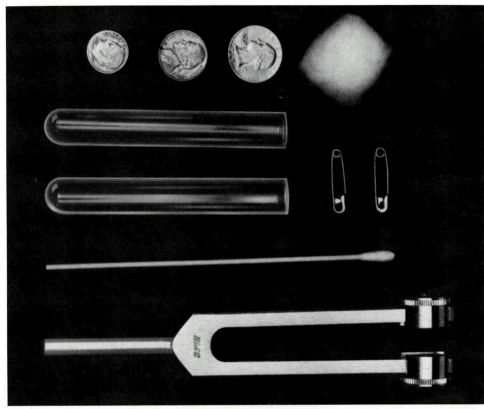

1 *Whenever you test a patient's sensory system, make sure she understands the examination procedure. She'll need reassurance that you won't hurt her. When you're sure she understands, tell her to close her eyes and keep them closed throughout the exam. Then proceed as follows:*

Gather this equipment: cotton, applicator stick or key, two safety pins, a tuning fork, two test tubes or small bottles, and three different sized coins (for example, a nickel, a dime, and a quarter).

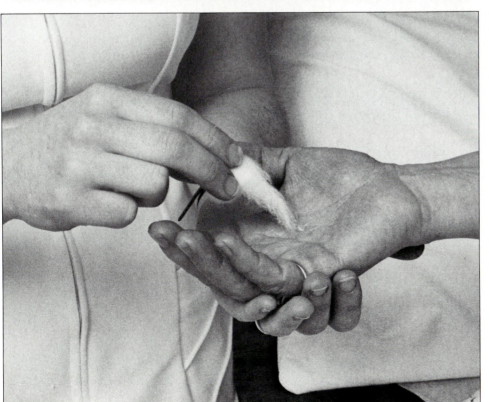

2 Now, ask your patient to extend her right arm in front of her. *Lightly* touch her right palm with a wisp of cotton, as the nurse is doing here. As you do this, instruct your patient to tell you when she feels something and what she feels.

Suppose your patient doesn't feel any sensation. Document the test result as *anesthesia on right palm.* If she perceives the touch as *lighter* than it is (less than normal sensation), document this as *hypoethesia on right palm.* If she perceives the touch as heavier than it is (greater than normal sensation), document this as *hyperethesia on right palm.*

Then, test her left palm and the other areas on her body, as explained on page 141. Be sure to refer to the dermatome chart on that page to locate and document specific areas of nerve sensation.

Nervous system

Testing your patient's sensory system continued

3 Next, test your patient's *pain* sensation. To do this, hold a pin loosely between your fingers. Lightly touch the pin's *point* to your patient's upper right arm, as shown here. Then, to maintain even pressure, slide your fingers down the pin, and *press* the point against her skin. Ask your patient to tell you when and where she feels any sensation.

[Inset] Next, touch the *blunt end* of the pin to your patient's arm, using the same technique as before. Ask your patient to describe the sensation exactly, including whether she feels the point or the blunt end of the pin.

Wait about 2 seconds, and repeat the test on your patient's left upper arm, her legs, and her torso. Remember to wait about 2 seconds between tests. Note your findings for each location.

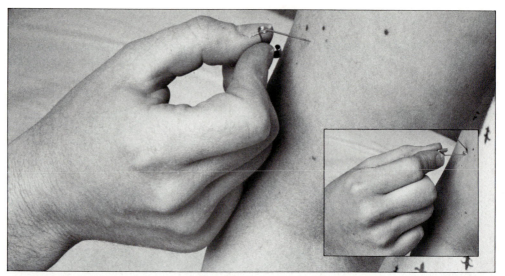

4 Now get ready to test your patient's hot/cold perception. To do this, fill one test tube (or bottle) with hot water and another test tube (or bottle) with cold water.

Then, touch the one filled with hot water to your patient's face. Hold it there for about 1 second. Then, touch the cold one to her face for about 1 second.

As you do, ask your patient to tell you what temperature she feels and where she feels it. Note any difficulty she has distinguishing hot from cold.

Using the same technique, alternately test her other body parts, varying test locations. Be sure to document test location, test performed, and the result.

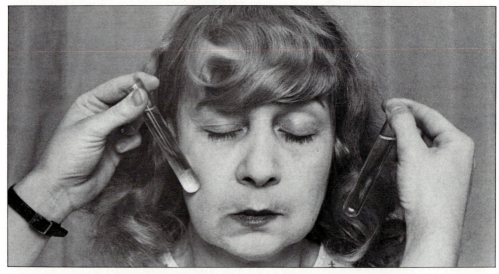

5 Now you're ready to test your patient's sensitivity to vibration. To do this, instruct your patient to block her ear canals with her index fingers. Place the base of a nonvibrating tuning fork against her right elbow, as the nurse is doing here.

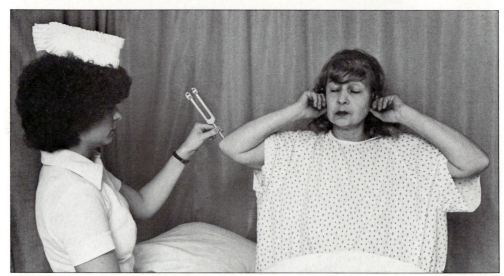

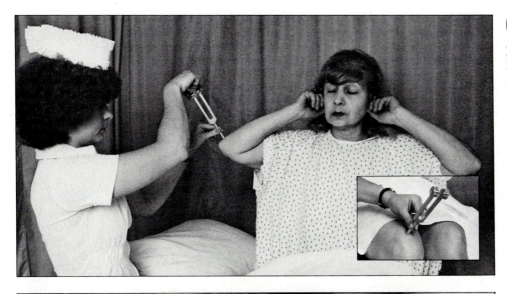

6 Vibrate the fork, then stop the vibration by placing your hand over the fork. Ask your patient to tell you when she feels the vibration start and stop. Obviously, you must stop the vibration before you remove the fork.

[Inset] Using the same procedure, test your patient's other elbow, her knees, and her ankles. Also test her sternum, ribs, clavicles, and spinous processes. Do your best to compare the vibration sensitivity on one side of her body to the other.

If you find an area where your patient's vibration sensitivity is deficient, repeat the test several times, to confirm your findings.

7 To test your patient's position sensitivity, hold her right index finger between your thumb and index finger. Ask your patient to tell you when she feels her finger being moved and in which direction.

Now, slowly move her finger up, as the nurse is doing here. Then move it down. If your patient has difficulty differentiating these directions, repeat the test on her right elbow and wrist. Remember to support her arm slightly above the joint being tested.

Using the same procedure, repeat the test on her left side.

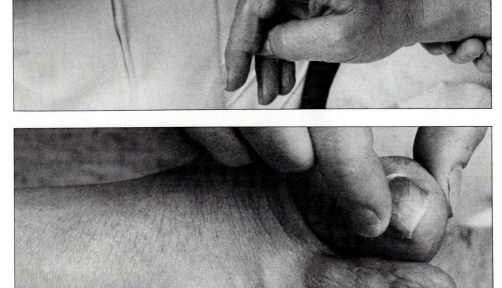

8 Perform the same test on her right big toe. Hold her toe between your right index finger and thumb.

Now, lift the toe up and then lower it. Ask your patient to tell you when she feels her toe being moved and in which direction. If your patient has difficulty differentiating these directions, repeat the test on her right ankle and knee.

Then, following the same procedure, test her left big toe.

Nervous system

Testing your patient's sensory system continued

9 Next, test your patient's sense of tactile discrimination. To do this, hold a pin in each hand. Following the guidelines in Step 2, use both pins to simultaneously prick your patient's right upper arm. Ask your patient to tell you what she feels, as well as when and where she feels it.

[Inset] Then, pinprick her right arm once. If everything's OK, she'll be able to differentiate one pinprick from two simultaneous pinpricks. Repeat the test with two pins, alternating the distance you hold the pins apart.

Repeat the test on your patient's legs and torso. Remember to document the kind of test performed, its location, and the result.

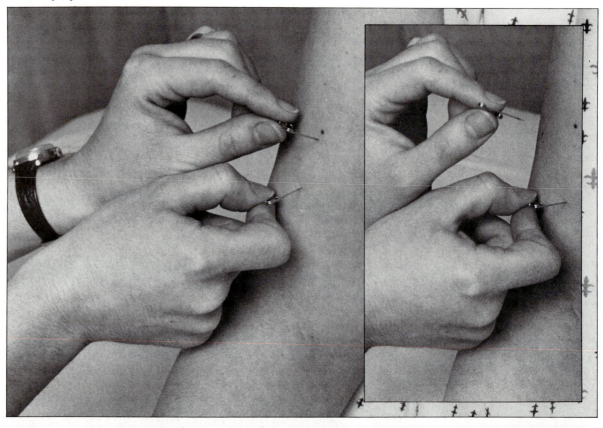

10 Now you're ready to assess your patient's extinction phenomenon, which is also part of the tactile discrimination test. Apply simultaneous fingertip pressure to comparable locations on your patient's arms. Then, alternately touch *just* your patient's right arm and *just* her left arm. As you do this, instruct your patient to tell you if she was touched on one or both arms. If she says both arms, consider this a normal response. If she says *one* arm, ask which one. Consider this an abnormal response.

Document the test performed, its location, and the result.

Repeat test on patient's trunk and legs.

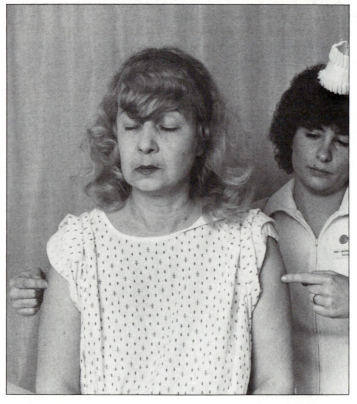

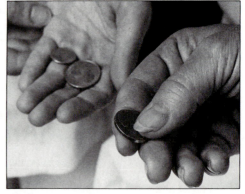

11 Finally, ask your patient to use her sense of touch to identify common objects; for example, a nickel, a dime, and a quarter.

To do this, put one coin in your patient's right hand. Then, ask her to identify it. Repeat with the other two coins, handing them to her one at a time. Repeat the test with her left hand.

Suppose she has difficulty identifying the coins. Repeat the test, using different objects; for example, a pen, a spoon, and a barrette.

Document the findings of all these tests in your nurses' notes.

How to use a dermatome chart

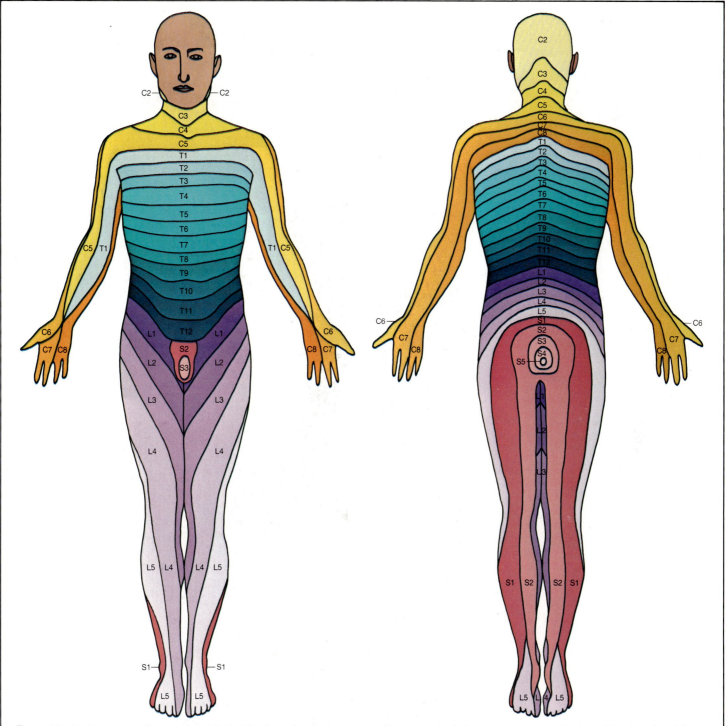

These illustrations show the segmental distribution of spinal nerves that transmit pain, temperature, and touch from the skin to the spinal cord.

As you assess your patient's sensory function, refer to this chart to document the specific areas tested, as well as the test results.

For example, let's assume your patient can't feel a pinprick on her right index and middle fingers. Using the dermatome chart properly, you'd document the test result as a loss of pain sensation in the C7 area.

Remember, you may find minor variations in the exact segmental levels, depending on the dermatome chart you're using.

Nervous system

Evaluating your patient's cranial nerves

The tests on the following pages will help you evaluate your patient's 12 cranial nerves. Study them carefully. But before you perform each test, explain the procedure to your patient. Document your findings in your nurses' notes.

Note: If you notice anything questionable, tell the doctor immediately.

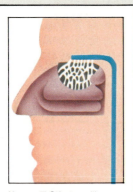

Nerve: ☐ Olfactory (I)

Type: Sensory

Function: Sense of smell

Test:
You'll need three substances with distinctive but familiar odors; for example, coffee, tobacco, and cloves. Ask your patient to close her eyes, and occlude her left nostril with her finger. Hold one of these substances under her right nostril, and ask her to identify the odor. Follow the same procedure with the other two substances. Then, repeat the entire test on her other nostril.

Normal findings:
Patient detects and correctly identifies all three odors.

Possible causes of abnormalities:
Temporary impairment from common cold; head trauma resulting in parosmia (perversion of sense of smell); compression of olfactory bulb by meningiomas or anterior fossa aneurysm; tumor infiltration in frontal lobe; or temporal lobe lesions, resulting in olfactory hallucinations

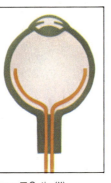

Nerve: ☐ Optic (II)

Type: Sensory

Function: Vision

Test: Visual acuity
Use a Snellen chart or an E chart to test your patient's visual acuity, as explained on pages 40 and 41.

Normal findings:
Corrected or uncorrected vision 20/20 or better

Test: Vision fields
Perform the test shown on pages 42 and 43.

Normal findings:
Patient's vision fields should be approximately the same as your own (provided your own vision is normal).

Test: Internal eye structure
Examine your patient's eyes with an ophthalmoscope, as explained on pages 36 and 37.

Normal findings:
Optic disc appears yellowish-pink and is round or oval, with clearly defined edges. Fundus appears uniformly orange, with optic disc located toward one side. Blood vessels extend outward from optic disc along borders of the fundus.

Possible causes of abnormalities:
Optic neuritis, toxic substances (for example, alcohol abuse), head trauma, chronic nephritis, diabetes mellitus, anemia, nutritional deficiencies, multiple sclerosis, chronic hypertension, intracranial tumors or aneurysms, or increased intracranial pressure

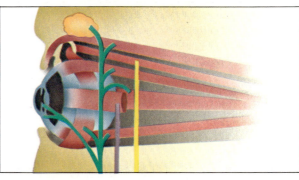

Nerves: ☐ Oculomotor (III); ☐ Trochlear (IV); ☐ Abducens (VI)

Type: Motor

Function:
Oculomotor: Innervates extrinsic eye muscles and ciliary muscle
Trochlear: Innervates superior oblique muscle
Abducens: Innervates external rectus muscle
Important: These three nerves operate as a unit and should be tested and evaluated together.

Test: Extrinsic eye muscles
Ask patient to open her eyes. Instruct her to focus on a point directly in front of her. Observe her ability to focus on one point effectively.

Normal findings:
Lower edges of lids meet bottom edges of irises; upper lids cover approximately 2 mm of irises.

Test: Direct pupillary response
Carefully note each pupil's size. Darken the room, and check your patient's eyes with a penlight. To do this, shine the light directly into one of your patient's pupils, as she keeps her other eye closed. Note the pupil's reaction. Then, check the other eye.

Normal findings:
Pupils constrict and remain constricted with light; pupils dilate when light is removed.

Test: Consensual pupillary response
Darken the room, but make sure your patient keeps both eyes open. Position the penlight directly in front of her right eye. Turn the penlight on, and observe the reaction of her left pupil. Then, check the other eye.

Normal findings:
Pupils constrict *bilaterally* and remain constricted with light.

Test: Extraocular eye movement
Follow the steps on page 39.

Normal findings:
Eyes move smoothly and bilaterally in all six cardinal fields of gaze.

Test: Accommodation and convergence
Follow guidelines on page 40.

Normal findings:
Both eyes converge on pencil at same level and distance. Patient maintains gaze on pencil when it's held 2'' to 3'' (5 to 7.6 cm) from the bridge of her nose. When your patient's eyes converge, both of her pupils constrict and remain constricted.

Abnormal findings in oculomotor (III) nerve damage:
Lid ptosis, with inability to completely open eye; eyeball deviated outward and slightly downward; pupil dilated and unreactive to light; nystagmus, and accommodation power lost

Abnormal findings in trochlear (IV) nerve damage:
Inability to turn eye downward or outward

Abnormal findings in abducens (VI) nerve damage:
Eyeball deviated inward, diplopia, paralysis of lateral gaze

Possible causes of abnormalities:
Trauma, multiple sclerosis, tumor or aneurysm at base of skull, increased intracranial pressure, botulism, or lead poisoning

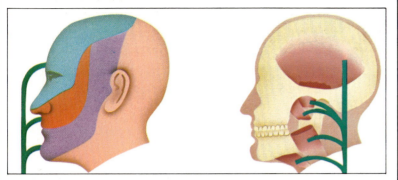

Nerve: ■ Trigeminal (V)

Types: Motor; sensory

Function: Chewing movements by innervation of masseter, temporal, and pterygoid muscles; corneal and sneezing reflexes; and sensations of face, scalp, and teeth

Test: Masseter muscle strength
 Instruct your patient to clench her teeth tightly. As she does, locate and palpate the masseter muscle bulges at her right and left jaw joints. Compare them.

Normal findings:
 Patient can clench teeth tightly. Masseter muscles bulge when teeth are clenched. On palpation, both masseter muscles feel equal in size and strength.

Test: Temporal muscle strength
 Instruct your patient to clench her teeth tightly. As she does, locate and palpate the temporal muscles at her temples. Compare them.

Normal findings:
 Patient can clench teeth tightly. On palpation, temporal muscles feel equal in size and strength.

Test: Pterygoid muscle strength
 Instruct your patient to clench her teeth. Ask your patient to resist your efforts to open her jaws. Then, grasp her lower jaw with one hand, and pull downward.

Normal findings:
 Patient keeps teeth tightly clenched, despite your efforts.

Test: Corneal reflex
 Instruct your patient to look up. Gently touch a cotton wisp to her right cornea. Repeat the test on her left cornea. *Note:* If your patient wears contact lenses, her corneal reflex may be diminished.

Normal findings:
 Patient blinks and her eyes tear when cornea's touched.

Test: Facial sensation
 Instruct your patient to close her eyes. Gently touch the point of a pin to one side of her forehead. Ask her to tell you *what* she feels, and *when* and *where* she feels it. Wait about 2 seconds, then repeat the test on the opposite side of her forehead.
 Next, repeat the test, using the blunt end of the pin. Finally, try the entire test (both ends of pin) on both sides of your patient's cheeks and jaw. Compare all findings.

Normal findings:
 Patient identifies the same sensation bilaterally, and tells when and where she feels it.

Test: Temperature sensation
 Follow the steps on page 138.

Normal findings:
 Patient identifies the same sensation bilaterally, and tells when and where she feels it.

Possible causes of abnormalities:
 Trauma, tic douloureux (trigeminal neuralgia), intracranial tumor, meningeal infection, intracranial aneurysm; when only descending tract is affected, syringobulbia (cavities in medulla oblongota) and multiple sclerosis. Also, pons lesion produces masticatory muscle paralysis and light touch sensation loss in face. Medulla lesion affecting descending tract causes pain and produces loss of temperature sensation and corneal reflex.

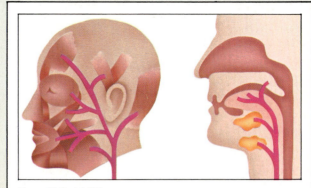

Nerve: ■ Facial (VII)

Type: Motor

Function: Facial expression, taste (anterior 2/3 of tongue), and salivary and lacrimal gland innervation

Test: Lower portion of facial nerve
 Observe your patient's face at rest and during conversation. Instruct her to purse her lips, smile, and frown.

Normal findings:
 Symmetrical facial contours, lines, wrinkles; symmetrical facial movement

Test: Lower portion of facial nerve
 Instruct your patient to puff out her cheeks and resist your efforts to collapse them.

Normal findings:
 Patient retains puffed cheeks despite your efforts to collapse them.

Test: Upper portion of facial nerve
 Ask your patient to close her eyes and resist your efforts to open them.

Normal findings:
 Patient resists efforts to open her eyes.

Test: Taste sensation on anterior 2/3 of tongue
 Wet cotton swabs in each of the following solutions: sugar (sweet), lemon juice (sour), saline (salty), quinine (bitter). Ask your patient to stick out her tongue. In turn, touch each swab to the front of her tongue, and ask her to identify the taste. Instruct your patient to rinse her mouth with water between tastes.

Normal findings:
 Patient correctly identifies sweet, sour, salty, and bitter tastes.
 Note: Remember, ability to taste may be inhibited by loss of sense of smell.

Possible causes of abnormalities:
 Trauma to peripheral nerve branches, mastoid surgery complications, temporal bone fracture, intracranial tumor or aneurysm, meningitis, herpes zoster, Paget's disease, or Bell's palsy

Nervous system

Evaluating your patient's cranial nerves continued

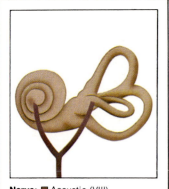

Nerve: ■ Acoustic (VIII)

Type: Sensory

Function: Hearing and sense of balance

Test: Air and bone conduction
Follow the steps shown on pages 50 and 51.

Normal findings:
Equal hearing in both ears. Air-conducted tone heard twice as long in both ears as bone-conducted tone.

Possible causes of abnormalities:
Inflammation; intracranial tumor; drug toxicity, particularly from aspirin, quinine, or streptomycin; middle fossa skull fracture

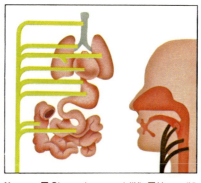

Nerves: ■ Glossopharyngeal (IX); ■ Vagus (X)

Types: Motor; sensory

Function: Swallowing movements and saliva secretion. Gag and swallow reflexes. Sensations in the pharynx and larynx, as well as taste on posterior 1/3 of tongue. Also, autonomic innervation of heart, lungs, esophagus, and stomach.
Important: These two nerves operate as a unit and should be tested and evaluated together.

Test: Throat movement
Instruct your patient to open her mouth and say *Ah*. As she does, observe her uvula and soft palate.

Normal findings:
When patient speaks, her uvula and soft palate move straight up.

Test: Gag reflex
Instruct your patient to open her mouth. As you depress her tongue with a tongue depressor, touch a cotton swab to either side of her pharynx.

Normal findings:
Patient gags. However, remember that a weak gag reflex may be normal in an elderly patient.

Test: Vocalization
Ask your patient to speak or cough.

Normal findings:
Patient's voice clear and strong. Cough strong.

Possible causes of glossopharyngeal (IX) nerve damage:
Intracranial tumors or infection

Possible causes of vagus (X) nerve damage:
Acute anterior poliomyelitis, intramedullary lesions; syringobulbia, vascular lesions, amyotrophic lateral sclerosis, multiple sclerosis

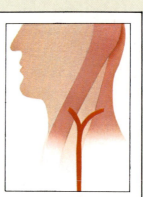

Nerve: ■ Spinal accessory (XI)

Type: Motor

Function: Innervates sterno-cleidomastoid and trapezius muscles

Test: Shoulder movement
Stand facing your patient. Place your hands on her shoulders. Ask her to lift her shoulders as you apply moderate downward pressure.

Normal findings:
Patient lifts shoulder despite your downward pressure.

Test: Neck muscle strength
Stand facing your patient. Place your left hand on the right side of your patient's face. Instruct her to turn her head toward her right side, against your hand's pressure. Repeat the procedure on the left side of her face.

Normal findings:
Firm jaw pressure against your hand

Possible causes of abnormalities:
Extramedullary tumors, occipital bone necrosis, inflammation, syringobulbia, amyotrophic lateral sclerosis, demyelinating diseases of the medulla

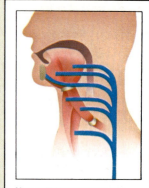

Nerve: ■ Hypoglossal (XII)

Type: Motor

Function: Innervates tongue muscle

Test: Tongue movement
Ask your patient to open her mouth, and observe her tongue at rest.

Normal findings:
Tongue is motionless and centered on mouth floor.

Test: Tongue movement
Instruct your patient to stick out her tongue.

Normal findings:
Protruding tongue appears centered between lips. Expect slight tongue movement.

Test: Tongue strength
Instruct your patient to press her tongue against one cheek wall. Apply fingertip pressure to outside of cheek as patient uses tongue to resist pressure. Repeat test on other cheek.

Normal findings:
Patient exerts firm tongue pressure against your fingertips.

Test: Tongue movement
Instruct your patient to dart her tongue in and out quickly. Then, ask her to stick her tongue out and move it from side to side as quickly as possible.

Normal findings:
Fast, smooth tongue movement

Possible causes of abnormalities:
Syringobulbia, amyotrophic lateral sclerosis, alcoholism, or CVA

How to test your patient's cerebellar function

1 *Are you testing your patient's cerebellar function? Perform the 10 tests outlined in this photostory, then consider all the results for your final evaluation.*

Begin as follows: First, ask your patient to walk heel to toe across the room. Observe her gait, noting posture, balance, and arm swing. Expect to see some side-to-side swaying.

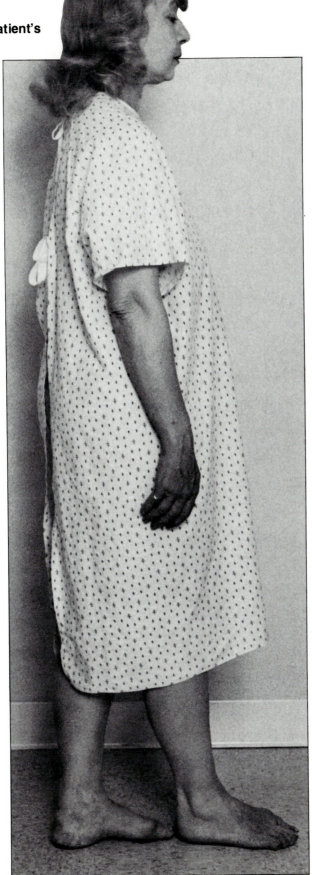

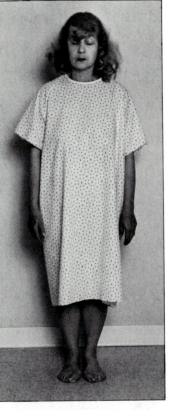

2 If you notice *excessive* swaying, your patient may have balance problems. To test her balance, perform the Romberg test.

First, ask your patient to stand with her feet together and her arms at her sides. Make sure her eyes are closed.

Observe your patient in this position for 1 minute. If everything's OK, you'll notice a slight side-to-side swaying. However, if you see excessive swaying (Romberg's sign), your patient may have a cerebellar dysfunction.

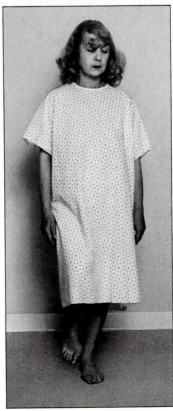

3 Suppose you observe the Romberg's sign. Continue your testing by asking your patient to hop on her right foot. Then, ask her to hop on her left foot. She should be able to maintain her balance on each foot. But remember, inability to maintain balance while hopping is not always a sign of cerebellar dysfunction. Some people can't hop because of arthritis or advanced age.

Nervous system

How to test your patient's cerebellar function continued

4 Now, seat your patient on the exam table, to test her arm and hand coordination.
   Instruct your patient to quickly and repeatedly pat her right thigh with her right hand. Note any difficulty she has doing this.
   Repeat the procedure with her left thigh and left hand.

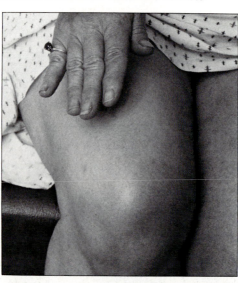

5 Next, ask your patient to alternately turn her right hand palm up (inset) and palm down as quickly as she can. Then, ask her to repeat the test with her left hand.

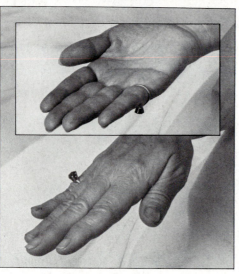

6 Tell your patient to sequentially touch her right thumb to each of her four fingers as quickly as she can.
   As before, ask her to repeat the test with her left hand.
   Note any problems.

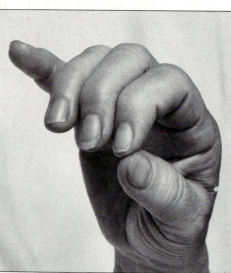

7 To test your patient's hand-eye coordination, position your right finger about 18" (45.7 cm) from your patient's face. Instruct your patient to alternately touch first your fingertip, then the *tip* of her nose, as fast as possible for 30 seconds (see inset). Note any difficulty she has making contact with either point.

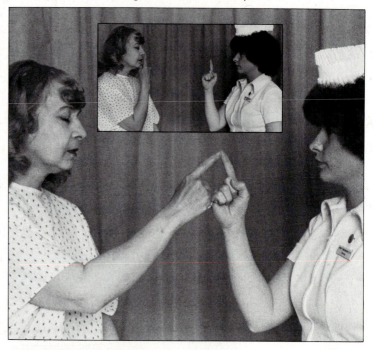

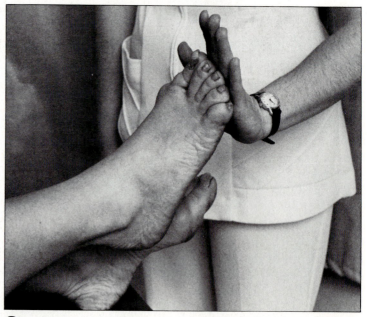

8 Now, ask your patient to lie on the exam table, and place a pillow under her head. Position yourself at the end of the table, facing your patient. Then, put your left hand about 4" (10 cm) from the ball of her right foot.
   Tell your patient to touch your hand with the ball of her foot. Does she have trouble following your order? Note it carefully.
   Repeat the same test on her left foot.

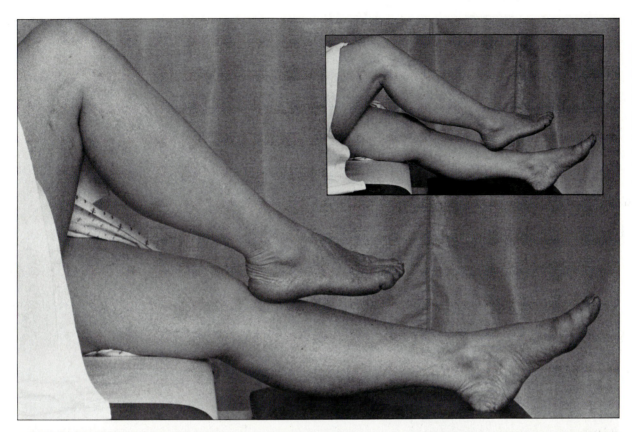

9 Instruct your patient first to place her right heel on her *left* knee, and then to slide her heel down her shin (see inset). Does she have any difficulty doing this? Note it. Have her repeat the test with her left heel and right knee.

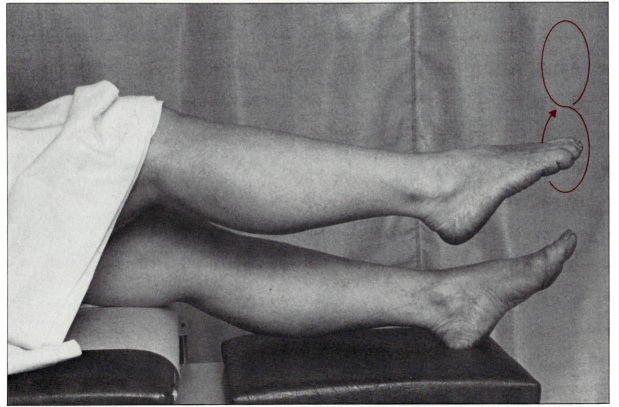

10 Finally, ask your patient to quickly and repeatedly draw an imaginary figure eight with her right big toe. Have her continue this process for 30 seconds. Then, ask her to repeat the test with her left big toe. Note any difficulties.
 When you've completed all 10 tests, document your findings in your nurses' notes.

Nervous system

How to test your patient's motor function

1 *Before you can accurately evaluate your patient's motor function, you must test the muscle strength in her wrists, fingers, arms, and legs. So you'll know exactly how to do this, we've photographed the steps here. Follow them carefully.* At the same time, inspect your patient for signs of muscle atrophy, involuntary tremors, and fasciculation.

Important: Never test a patient's muscle strength if you have any muscle weakness yourself. If you do, the test results will be inaccurate.

Here's how to perform the tests. First, explain the testing procedure to your patient, and answer any questions she may have. Then, ask her to stand in front of you with her eyes closed. Extend her arms, with her palms up.

Instruct her to maintain this position for 30 seconds. During this time, note any tendency she has to turn her palms downward (pronation), lower her arms, or bend her arms at the elbows. Also, note any tremors or involuntary movements. Any difficulty your patient has may indicate muscle weakness.

Remember: If muscle weakness is greater in the distal joints, it may indicate a neurologic disorder.

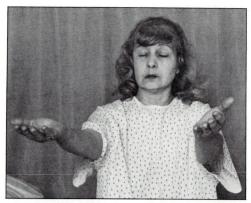

2 Now, tell your patient to open her eyes. Instruct her to extend her arms at shoulder level in front of her. Turn her palms downward. Then, ask her to maintain this position.

Now, position yourself at your patient's right side. Place your hands on her wrists, and try to push her arms downward, as the nurse is doing here. As you do this, observe your patient's shoulder blades. If you notice the tips of the blades protruding abnormally, suspect a serratus anterior muscle weakness.

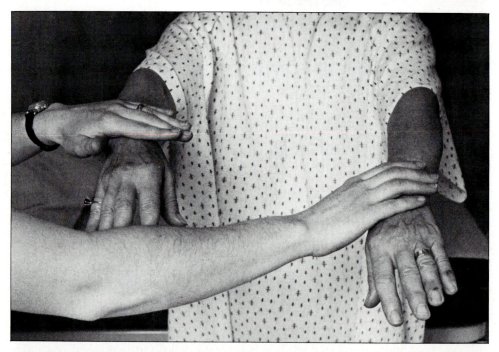

3 Ask your patient to close her eyes and to extend both arms above her head. Position her palms so they're facing forward. Then, instruct her to hold this position for 30 seconds. As she does, note any downward drifting of her arms or hands. If you see any, suspect hemiparesis or shoulder-girdle muscle weakness.

[Inset] While your patient maintains this position, step behind her. Now, place your hands on both her wrists, as shown, and alternately push down on each one. Describe each arm's strength.

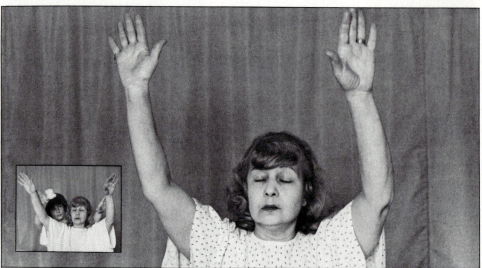

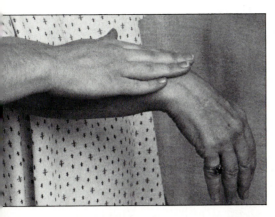

4 Now, face your patient again. Instruct her to hold her right arm at her side, with her elbow *flexed* and her forearm *extended forward,* as shown here. Place your hand on her wrist, and try to move her arm up, then down. Describe the strength of her arm.

Repeat the test on her left arm.

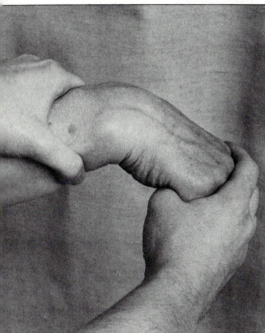

5 Now test your patient's forearm and finger strength, and her radial and ulnar nerve function. To do this, instruct your patient to remain standing and to keep her right arm flexed. Place your left hand on her forearm, just behind her wrist. Put your right hand as shown. Explain that you'll be pressing *down* on her hand and ask her to resist.

Start exerting downward pressure. If your patient's wrist bends easily, she may have a radial nerve disorder. Note this carefully.

Repeat the procedure on her left arm.

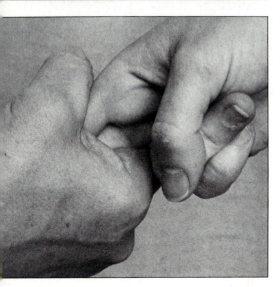

6 Next, place your thumb on top of your ring and little fingers. Then, ask your patient to grasp your fingers as tightly as possible with her right hand.

As she does, try to pull your fingers out of her grip. If her forearm muscle strength is adequate, you'll have difficulty pulling your fingers loose.

Repeat the procedure with her left hand.

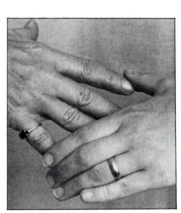

7 Now, tell your patient to spread the fingers of her right hand and to resist your pressure against them. Grasp her hand with your left index finger against her little finger and your thumb against her index finger, as shown here. Squeeze her fingers as tightly as possible. If all's well, you'll have trouble doing this. If her fingers seem weak, suspect an ulnar nerve disorder.

Repeat the procedure on her left hand.

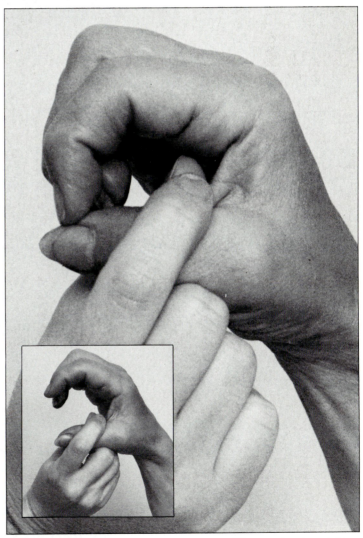

8 Instruct your patient to press her right thumb against her right fingertips. Then, tell her to resist your efforts to separate them. Hook your thumb and index finger through her fingers.

[Inset] Now, try to pull her thumb and fingers apart, as shown here. Note any weakness.

Repeat the procedure on her left hand.

Nervous system

How to test your patient's motor function continued

9 Now you're ready to test your patient's leg strength. Position your patient flat on her back on the exam table. With one hand, press down on her right knee as you instruct her to elevate her leg. Note any problems she has doing so.

Repeat the procedure on her left leg.

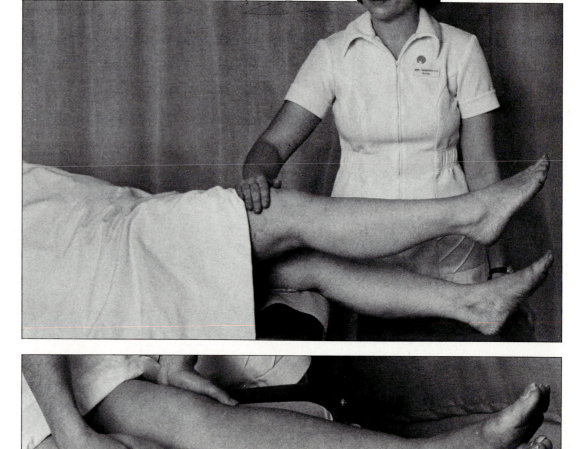

10 Now, press the outside of her legs together at the knees. Instruct her to attempt spreading her legs apart, against your pressure. Note any difficulty.

11 Next, remove your hands, and tell your patient to spread her legs slightly apart. Press your right hand on the inside of her right knee and your left hand on the inside of her left knee. Instruct her to attempt bringing her legs together, as you apply outward pressure. Again, note any difficulties she has.

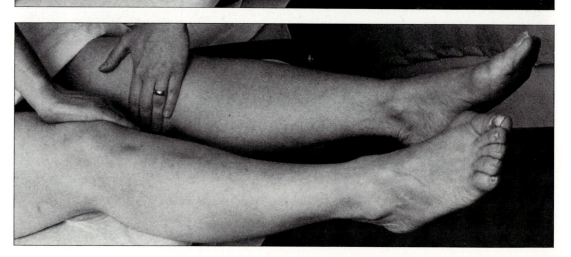

12 Now, ask your patient to flex her right leg at the knee, and to put her foot flat on the exam table. Place your right hand on your patient's raised knee and put your left hand over her right Achilles tendon, as shown here. Instruct her to resist your pressure. Then attempt to straighten her leg by using your left hand to pull her foot outward as you press down on her knee.

Repeat the test on her left leg.

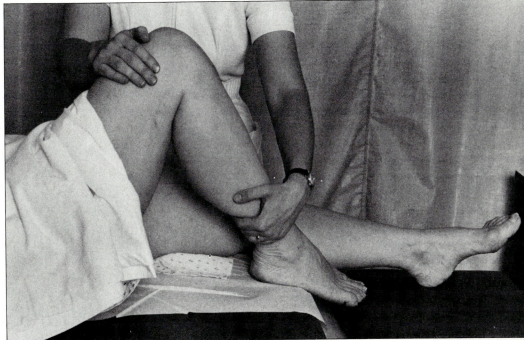

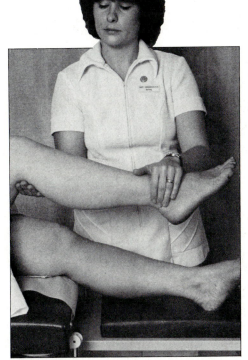

13 Remove your hands, and tell your patient to extend both her legs flat on the exam table. Then, ask her to raise her right foot off the table.

Place one hand under her right knee and your other hand on her ankle. Then, try to push her foot down on the table. At the same time, instruct her to resist your pressure.

Repeat the procedure on your patient's left leg.

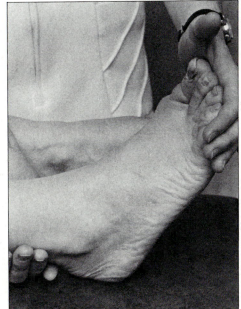

14 Once again, ask your patient to extend both legs flat on the exam table, with her toes pointing upward. Place one hand under her right ankle and your other hand on the ball of her right foot, as the nurse is doing here.

Then, push against her right foot, so it flexes toward her knee. Ask your patient to resist your pressure.

Repeat the procedure on her left foot.

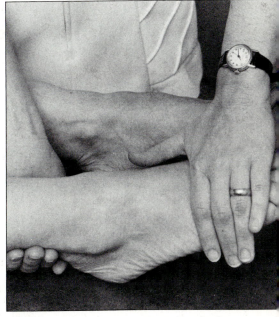

15 Finally, keeping one hand under her right ankle, place your other hand on top of her foot.

Then, try to flex her foot down. Ask your patient to resist your pressure.

Repeat the procedure on her left foot.

When you've completed these tests, document any evidence of muscle weakness, atrophy, or tremors, in your nurses' notes.

Nervous system

Evaluating your patient's motor responses: Muscle tone

1 *To do a thorough examination of your patient, you'll need to evaluate her muscle tone. Begin by explaining the exam procedure to your patient.*

Observe all her muscles, noting any abnormal movement, such as rapid and continuous twitching, tremors, tics, rapid and jerky movements (chorea), and athetosis.

Now, measure the muscles in your patient's upper right arm, as the nurse is doing here. Then, measure the muscles in her upper left arm. Compare both measurements, noting any differences. Record for future comparison.

Also, measure the muscles in the widest part of her thighs and calves, and note any differences.

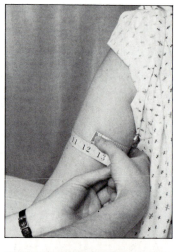

2 Tell your patient to relax, as you support her right elbow with one hand. Now, with your other hand, grasp her wrist, and bring her arm through a complete range of motion. Note any flaccidity, pain, rigidity, jerking, spasticity, or resistance.

Repeat the procedure with her left arm.

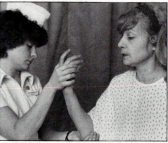

3 While you support your patient's right knee with one hand, position your other hand under her heel. Bring her leg through a complete range of motion. Again, note any flaccidity, pain, rigidity, jerking, spasticity, or resistance.

Repeat the procedure with her left leg.

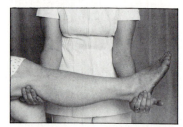

4 What if you observe abnormal movement in your patient's arms or legs? Perform the following tests:

First, tell your patient to sit on the exam table, with her legs dangling. Support her heels with the palms of your hands. Lift her heels to knee level, as shown here.

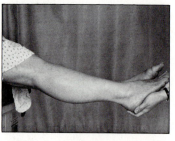

5 Remove your palms from her heels. Observe your patient's leg movement.

If everything's OK, her legs will swing freely. However, suppose your patient's legs swing only slightly or not at all. Note the degree of rigidity and document it.

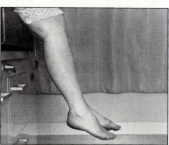

6 Next, ask your patient to keep her right arm loose, as you position your hand slightly above her wrist. Shake her arm several times, noting the wrist movement. If all's well, her wrist will move freely. Note any abnormalities.

Repeat the procedure on her left arm.

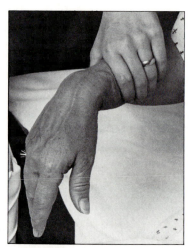

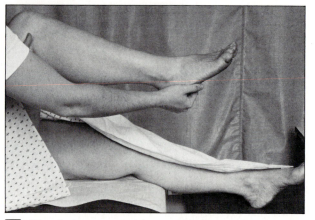

7 Now, instruct your patient to lie flat on the exam table. Position one hand under her right knee. Place the palm of your other hand under her right heel, and lift her foot 12" (30 cm) off the table.

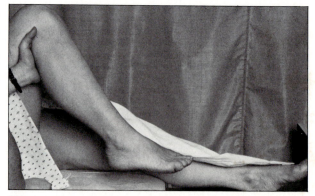

8 Keeping one hand under her knee, remove your palm from her heel. Her foot should fall quickly and freely. If her leg remains extended or falls slowly, she may have rigidity or spasticity.

Repeat the procedure on her left leg.

Finally, document all your findings in your nurses' notes.

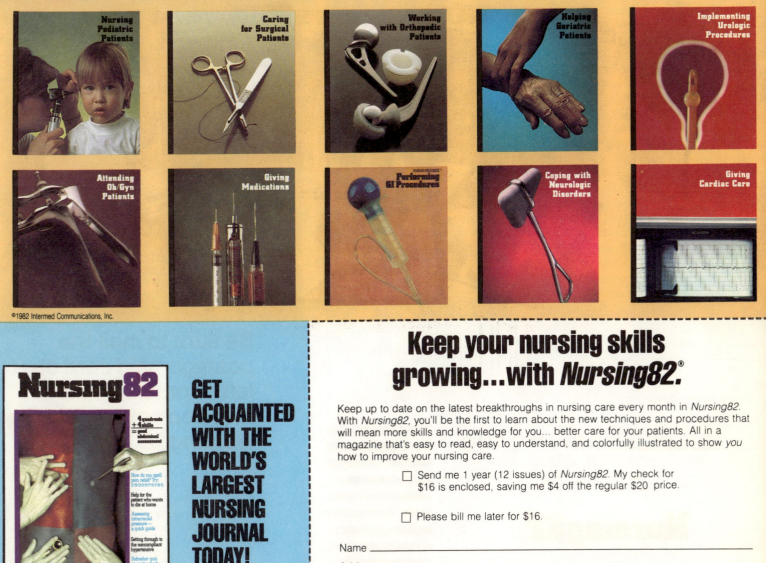

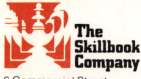
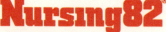

Identifying nervous system disorders

Assessment variables	Cerebrovascular accident (CVA), with occlusion of left middle cerebral artery	Early cerebral edema from head injury	Parkinson's disease	Spinal fracture, with complete transection at C6 level	Early acute septic meningitis
Pain	• Frontal headache. (If patient's conscious but can't speak clearly, he may show pain by pointing to forehead.)	• Can't communicate pain	• None	• Localized neck pain	• Severe headache • Neck pain
Eye exam (visual acuity, pupillary response, and ophthalmoscopy)	• Right half of vision field lost in each eye. • Pupils are equal in size and react to light. • Flame-shaped hemorrhages in the retina	• In early stages, no characteristic changes	• No characteristic changes	• No characteristic changes	• No characteristic changes
Motor function examination	• Drooping mouth on right side • Right-sided partial paralysis (hemiparesis) • Muscle strength and movement unaffected on left side.	• Symmetrical deep tendon reflexes • Painful stimuli on face causes bilateral, symmetrical, facial movement. • Fingertip pressure on supraorbital structure causes symmetrical withdrawal of all extremities.	• Slow body movements and slow, shuffling gait • Arm, leg, and neck rigidity • Pill-rolling hand tremor • Mask-like facial expression	• Spontaneous breathing • Loss of voluntary body movement below shoulders • Constant, spastic elbow flexion	• Patient exhibits purposeless movement; for example, plucking at the bed sheet. • Patient can move all extremities. • Restlessness
Sensory function examination	• Right-sided loss of superficial sensation	• No verbal response to sensory function tests, because patient is unconscious. For his motor responses to these tests, see the last two entries above.	• No characteristic changes	• No sensation below anterior clavicles or tops of posterior scapulae • Sensation on upper third of arms, from shoulders to thumbs	• No characteristic changes
Mental status	• Patient oriented to person, place, and time. (If he's conscious but can't speak clearly, he may respond appropriately to questions by nodding or shaking his head.)	• Patient responds to verbal stimuli by opening his eyes but can't follow commands.	• Patient alert and oriented	• Patient oriented to person, place, and time	• Increasing irritability • Verbally abusive • Patient oriented to person; disoriented to time and place. • Patient can follow simple commands.
Special	• Normal temperature and respirations • Rapid, regular pulse • Slurred, incomprehensible speech	• Normal respirations • Visible signs of head injury; for example, forehead or scalp lacerations • Possible skull fracture	• Profuse sweating • Seborrhea • Speech rapid, low, and monotonous • Depression	• Postural hypotension	• Positive Kernig's sign. (To test for this, place patient on back. Flex his leg at hip and knee, then straighten knee. Signs of pain or resistance indicate meningeal inflammation.) • Positive Brudzinki sign. (To test, place patient on back. Put your hands behind his head and flex his neck forward. Signs of pain, resistance, hip or knee flexion suggest meningeal inflammation.)

DOCUMENTING

NURSING DATA BASE
(Assessment)

SECTION I: Date _12/18/80_   Time _1:30 P.M._   Name _Marilyn Copeland_

Mode _admitted ambulatory_   Age _54_

T _98.8_ P _84_ R _18_ BP _136/78_ Ht _5'4"_ Wt _142 lbs._

Diet _House_   Bloodwork: Yes _X_ No ___   Urinalysis: Yes _X_ No ___

Prosthesis: Glasses ⌐ Contact lenses ⌐ Dentures ⌐ Hearing aids ⌐ Other ⌐

Ambulation aids: Walker ⌐ Cane ⌐ Crutches ⌐ Wheelchair ⌐

General orientation to hospital environment by: _Mary H. Obenrader, RN_   _12/18/80_
                                                    Signature   Date

Section I must be completed and signed by an RN or LPN on all admissions.

SECTION II: Date _12/18/80_   Time _2:00 P.M._

Reason for hospitalization or chief complaint: _"dizzy spells several times a day"_

Duration of this problem/onset: _onset Nov. 28th-increasing in severity during past week_

Admitting diagnosis: _vertigo-unknown etiology_

Previous hospitalizations and illnesses:

Date	Doctor	Where	Type of illness or surgery and reaction
3/56	Dr. James Osborn	St. Francis Hosp., NYC	Tonsillectomy
5/65	Dr. Samuel Clark	Phila. G. Hosp, Phila, PA	Fracture Ⓡ radius

Allergies (what and type of reaction) _Penicillin - severe rash, Pollens-sneezing, itchy eyes._

Immunization: DPT _?_ Polio _?_ TB _7/78_ (Reaction _neg (Tine)_)

Measles _had disease_ Mumps _had disease_ Rubella _had disease_

Medications code: A—Sent home with family; B—May be self-administered; C—Not brought in with patient.

Name	Code	Dose and time	Time of last dose	Patient's understanding of purpose
Benadryl	C	25mg ℗ Q.I.D. PRN	Sept. 1980	Takes drug for allergy

Social history of alcohol _occasional social_ Smoking _Smoked from age 18 to 40. Has not smoked in 14 yrs._

Family Health History:

Diabetes _none_ Heart _father_ Cancer _uterine maternal grandmother_ Kidney _none_ T.B. _none_ COPD _none_

Asthma _none_ Epilepsy _none_ Psychiatric _none_ Other _____

Review of Systems:

EENT _Vision 20/40 Ⓡ eye - 20/20 Ⓛ eye; Eyes unable to converge and accommodate properly; eardrum-pearl gray-no inflammation; nose-no drainage; sinuses illuminate well; poor oral hygiene-many teeth missing-remaining in poor condition._

Neurologic _muscle strength normal; difficulty c̄ fine motor coordination._

Respiratory *Chest-normal shape; lungs clear; occasional nonproductive cough*

Cardiovascular *Heart sounds clear; rate 80 to 84; rhythm normal; aortic pulsation seen above umbilicus.*

GI *rounded abd; bowel sounds normal; liver normal size.*

GU *Kidneys nonpalpable, nontender.*

Skin *warm and dry; no rashes or bruises; ® breast larger than left-no lumps or masses.*

Extremities *all peripheral pulses present and strong.*

Mental/emotional status *Affect appears flat; very little change of expression.*

Reproductive *Bimanual vaginal palpation-normal; ovaries somewhat atrophied; vaginal walls pink; stellate cervical as; swabs taken for cytology and gonococcal smear.*

Signature *Mary H. Obenrader, RN*

Section II must be completed and signed by an RN (Sections I and II must be completed on short-term admissions).

SECTION III: Date *12/18/80*   Time *2 P.M.*

Occupation: *Part-time secretary; housewife*

Family structure: *Husband; 2 sons 1 daughter-all married living away from home*

Family responsibilities: *Husband can manage alone.*

Language spoken: *English*

Patterns:

Hygiene *Showers every other day*

Rest/sleep *retires at 10 P.M. Usually wakes several times a night to urinate.*

Activity status *Daily walk-no other regular exercise*

Elimination habits *Voids frequently and has nocturia; BM daily; occasional laxative.*

Meals/diet *no special diet; dislikes lamb and green beans*

Health practices *Needs to see a dentist*

Typical daily profile: *7 AM to 12 noon housework; secretarial work 3 afternoons a week; does needlepoint in spare time.*

Information obtained from: Patient *X* Family ____ Previous records ____

COMMENTS: *Well-developed; slightly obese female in no acute distress at this time.*

Signature *Mary H. Obenrader, RN*

Section III—Completed by an RN. (Sections I, II and III must be completed on all patients except those defined by policy as short-term.)

Selected references

Books

Andreoli, Kathleen G., et al. COMPREHENSIVE CARDIAC CARE, 4th ed. St. Louis: C.V. Mosby Co., 1979.

ASSESSING VITAL FUNCTIONS ACCURATELY. Nursing Skillbook® Series. Springhouse, Pa.: Intermed Communications, Inc., 1977.

Barr, Murray L. THE HUMAN NERVOUS SYSTEM: AN ANATOMICAL VIEW POINT, 2nd ed. New York: Harper & Row Publishers, Inc., 1973.

Bates, Barbara. A GUIDE TO PHYSICAL EXAMINATION, 2nd ed. Philadelphia: J.B. Lippincott Co., 1979.

Benchimol, Alberto. NON-INVASIVE TECHNIQUES IN CARDIOLOGY. Baltimore: Williams & Wilkins Co., 1977.

Berkow, Robert, and John H. Talbott. THE MERCK MANUAL OF DIAGNOSIS AND THERAPY. Rahway, N.J.: Merck & Co., Inc. 1977.

Beyers, Marjorie, and Susan Dudas. THE CLINICAL PRACTICE OF MEDICAL-SURGICAL NURSING. Boston: Little, Brown & Co., 1977.

Boies, L. FUNDAMENTALS OF OTOLARYNGOLOGY, 5th ed. Philadelphia: W.B. Saunders Co., 1978.

Bower, Fay L., and Robinetta Wheeler. NURSING ASSESSMENT. New York: John Wiley & Sons, 1977.

Brunner, Lillian S., and Doris S. Suddarth. THE LIPPINCOTT MANUAL OF NURSING PRACTICE. Philadelphia: J.B. Lippincott Co., 1974.

Burns, Kenneth R., and Patricia J. Johnson. HEALTH ASSESSMENT IN CLINICAL PRACTICE. Englewood Cliffs, N.J.: Prentice-Hall, Inc., 1980.

Buckingham, William B., et al. PRIMER OF CLINICAL DIAGNOSIS. New York: Harper & Row Publishers, Inc., 1971.

Campbell, Claire. NURSING DIAGNOSIS AND INTERVENTION IN NURSING PRACTICE. New York: John Wiley & Sons, 1978.

Campbell, Meredith F., and J. Hartwell Harrison. UROLOGY, vol. 1. Philadelphia: W.B. Saunders Co., 1978.

Chusid, Joseph G. CORRELATIVE NEUROANATOMY AND FUNCTIONAL NEUROLOGY, 16th ed. Los Altos, Calif.: Lange Medical Publications, 1976.

Cope, Zachary. THE EARLY DIAGNOSIS OF THE ACUTE ABDOMEN, 14th ed. New York: Oxford University Press, 1972.

COPING WITH NEUROLOGIC PROBLEMS PROFICIENTLY. Nursing Skillbook® Series. Springhouse, Pa.: Intermed Communications, Inc., 1979.

Degowin, Elmer, and Richard L. Degowin. BEDSIDE DIAGNOSTIC EXAMINATION. New York: Macmillan Publishing Co., Inc., 1976.

Degowin, Elmer, and Richard L. Degowin. DIAGNOSTIC EXAMINATION. London: The MacMillan Company, 1979.

DOCUMENTING PATIENT CARE RESPONSIBLY. Nursing Skillbook® Series. Springhouse, Pa.: Intermed Communications, Inc., 1978.

Fowkes, William C., Jr., and Virginia K. Hunn. CLINICAL ASSESSMENT FOR THE NURSE PRACTITIONER. St. Louis: C.V. Mosby Co., 1973.

Fuerst, Elinor V., et al. FUNDAMENTALS OF NURSING: THE HUMANITIES AND THE SCIENCES IN NURSING, 5th ed. Philadelphia: J.B. Lippincott Co., 1974.

Guyton, Arthur C. TEXTBOOK OF MEDICAL PHYSIOLOGY, 5th ed. Philadelphia: W.B. Saunders Co., 1976.

Hall, Ian S., and Bernard H. Colman. DISEASES OF THE NOSE, THROAT, AND EAR, 11th ed. New York: Longman Inc., 1976.

Harvey, A. McGehee, and Richard J. Johns. THE PRINCIPLES AND PRACTICE OF MEDICINE. New York: Appleton-Century-Crofts, 1972.

Havener, William H. SYNOPSIS OF OPHTHALMOLOGY, 4th ed. St. Louis: C.V. Mosby Co., 1975.

Judge, Richard D., and George D. Zuidema, eds. METHODS OF CLINICAL EXAMINATION: A PHYSIOLOGIC APPROACH, 3rd ed. Boston: Little, Brown & Co., 1974.

Keeney, Arthur H. OCULAR EXAMINATION: BASIS AND TECHNIQUES. St. Louis: C.V. Mosby Co., 1970.

Acknowledgements

Kingsley, Benedict, et al. ADVANCES IN NON-INVASIVE DIAGNOSTIC TESTING OF CARDIAC PATIENTS. Thorofare, N.J.: Charles B. Slack, Inc., 1975.

Kintzel, Kay C., et al. ADVANCED CONCEPTS IN CLINICAL NURSING, 2nd ed. Philadelphia: J.B. Lippincott Co., 1977.

Luckmann, Joan, and Karen C. Sorensen. MEDICAL-SURGICAL NURSING: A PSYCHOPHYSIOLOGIC APPROACH. Philadelphia: W.B. Saunders Co., 1974.

Morgan, William L., and George L. Engel. CLINICAL APPROACH TO THE PATIENT. Philadelphia: W.B. Saunders Co., 1969.

Newby, Hayes A. AUDIOLOGY, 3rd ed. Englewood Cliffs, N.J.: Prentice-Hall, Inc., 1972.

Pracy, R., et al. A SHORT TEXTBOOK: EAR, NOSE, AND THROAT, 2nd ed. Philadelphia: J.B. Lippincott Co., 1975.

Prior, John A., and Jack S. Silberstein. PHYSICAL DIAGNOSIS: THE HISTORY AND EXAMINATION OF THE PATIENT, 5th ed. St. Louis: C.V. Mosby Co., 1977.

PROVIDING RESPIRATORY CARE. Nursing Photobook™ Series. Springhouse, Pa.: Intermed Communications, Inc., 1979.

Robbins, Stanley L. PATHOLOGIC BASIS OF DISEASE. Philadelphia: W.B. Saunders Co., 1974.

Sauve, Mary J., and Angela Pecherer. CONCEPTS AND SKILLS IN PHYSICAL ASSESSMENT. Philadelphia: W.B. Saunders Co., 1977.

Selkurt, Ewald E. PHYSIOLOGY, 4th ed. Boston: Little, Brown & Co., 1976.

Sherman, Jacques L., Jr., and Sylvia K. Fields, eds. GUIDE TO PATIENT EVALUATION. Flushing, N.Y.: Medical Examination Publishing Co., 1978.

Thorn, George W., et al, eds. HARRISON'S PRINCIPLES OF INTERNAL MEDICINE, 8th ed. New York: McGraw-Hill Book Co., 1977.

Vaughan, Daniel, and Taylor Asbury. GENERAL OPHTHALMOLOGY, 8th ed. Los Altos, Calif.: Lange Medical Publications, 1974.

Watson, Jeanette E. MEDICAL-SURGICAL NURSING AND RELATED PHYSIOLOGY. Philadelphia: W.B. Saunders Co., 1972.

Wilson, Robert Francis., ed. CRITICAL CARE MANUAL: PRINCIPLES AND TECHNIQUES OF CRITICAL CARE. Kalamazoo, Mich.: Upjohn Co., 1976.

Winter, Chester, C., and Marilyn R. Barker. NURSING CARE OF PATIENTS WITH UROLOGIC DISEASES, 3rd ed. St. Louis: C.V. Mosby Co., 1972.

Periodicals

Keithley, Joyce K. *Proper Nutritional Assessment Can Prevent Hospital Malnutrition,* NURSING79. 9:68-72.

Mechner, Francis. *Patient Assessment: Examination of the Eye,* Part II, AMERICAN JOURNAL OF NURSING. January 1975.

Mechner, Francis. *Patient Assessment: Neurological Examination,* Part I, AMERICAN JOURNAL OF NURSING. September 1975.

Mechner, Francis. *Patient Assessment: Neurological Examination,* Part III, AMERICAN JOURNAL OF NURSING. April 1976.

Pegues, Thelma. *Assessment of the Black Patient,* CRITICAL CARE UPDATE. 6:10:25-32, October 1979.

Snyder, Mariah, and Rebecca Baum. *Assessing Station and Gait,* AMERICAN JOURNAL OF NURSING. July 1974, pp. 1256-1257.

Stoll, Ruth I. *Guidelines for Spiritual Assessment,* AMERICAN JOURNAL OF NURSING. September 1979, pp. 1574-1578.

We'd like to thank the following people and companies for their help with this PHOTOBOOK:

Brian Altman, MD
Pediatric Ophthalmology
Abington, Pa.

ATCO SURGICAL CO.
Division of Amasia Trading Co., Inc.
New York, N.Y.
Syed N. Shamsi, President

G. Richard Bennett, MS, OD
The Eye Institute
Pennsylvania College of Optometry
Philadelphia, Pa.

DELCREST MEDICAL PRODUCTS & SERVICES CO.
Philadelphia, Pa.

Karen Lit, CO

WELCH ALLYN, INC.
Skaneateles Falls, N.Y.
Donald E. Plath,
Marketing Manager

Also the staff of:

MONTGOMERY HOSPITAL
Norristown, Pa.

Index

Index